WHOLE
NEW YOU

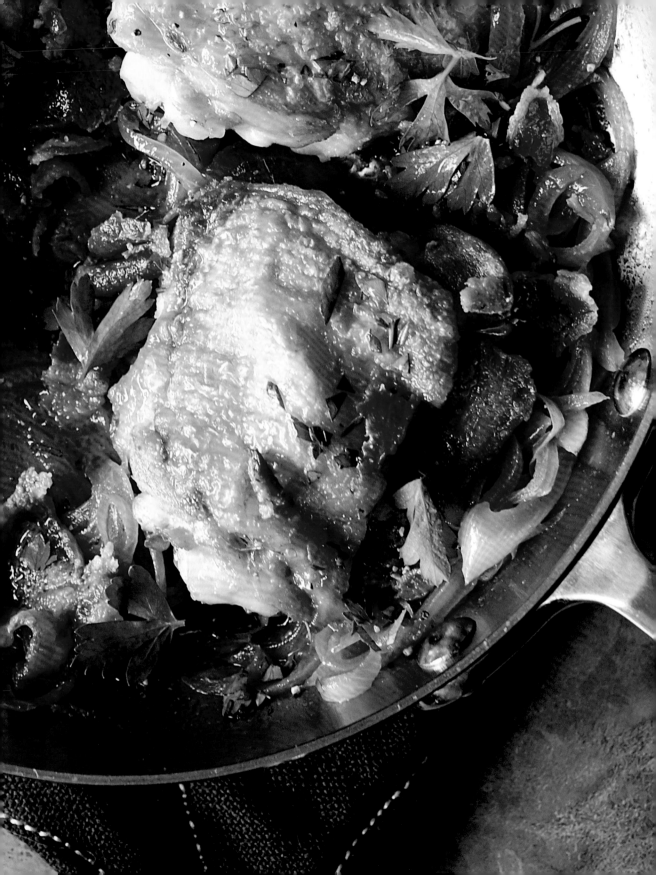

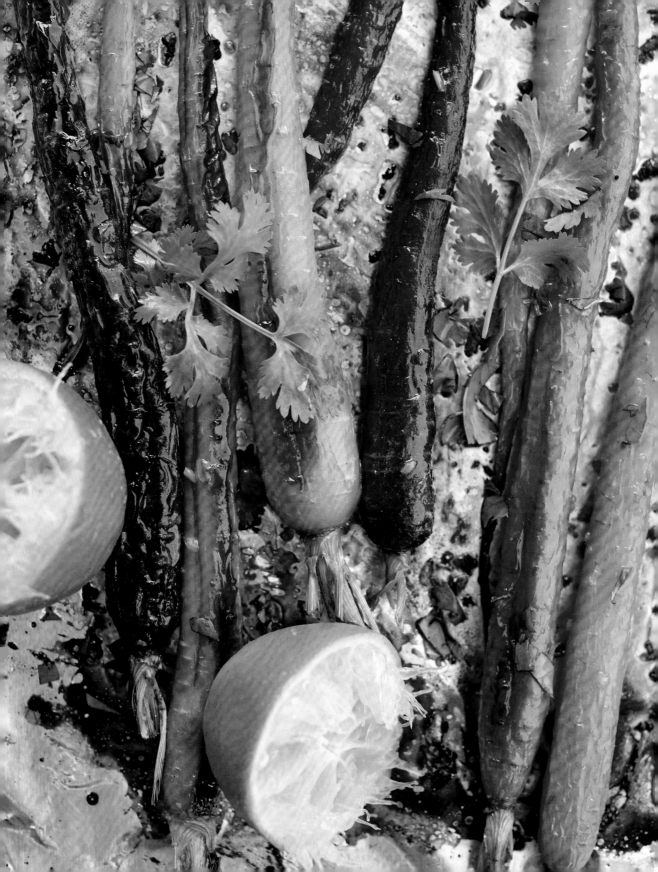

by Tia Mowry

———

WHOLE NEW YOU

OH, BABY!

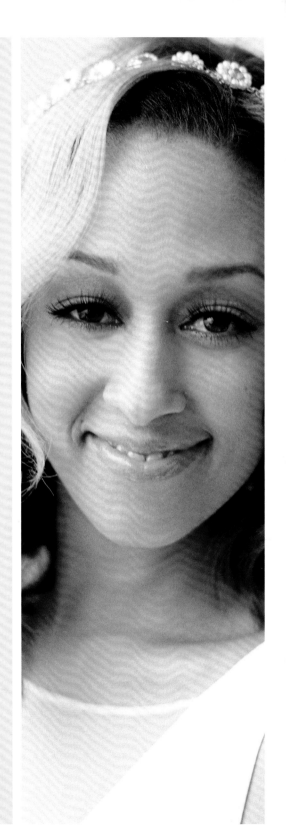

WHOLE
NEW YOU

HOW REAL FOOD
TRANSFORMS YOUR LIFE,
FOR A HEALTHIER,
MORE GORGEOUS YOU

TIA
MOWRY

with *Jessica Porter*

BALLANTINE BOOKS

NEW YORK

Copyright © 2017 by Tia Mowry-Hardrict

Published in the United States by Ballantine Books,
an imprint of Random House, a division of
Penguin Random House LLC, New York.

BALLANTINE and the HOUSE colophon are registered trademarks
of Penguin Random House LLC.

ISBN 978-1-101-96735-5
ebook ISBN 978-1-101-96737-9

Photos on pages xiv, 69, 74, 89, 90, 298 are courtesy of the author.
Photos on pages v, vii, 2, 7, 11, 22, 92 are © Elizabeth Messina.
All remaining photos are © Jennifer Davick.

Printed in China

randomhousebooks.com

987654321

First Edition

Book design by Barbara M. Bachman

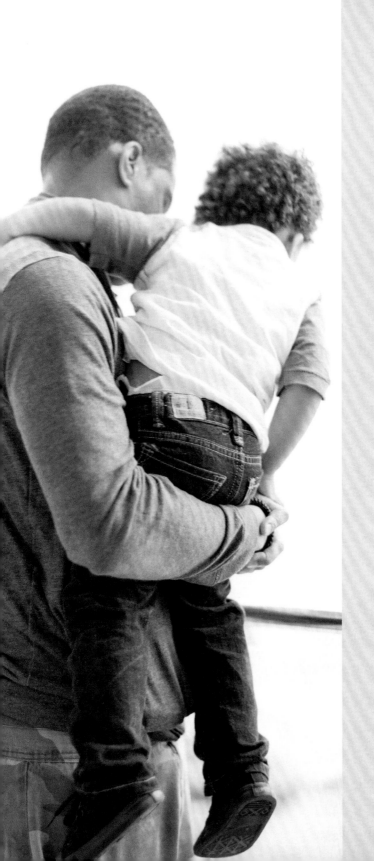

This book is dedicated to my husband, Cory, and our incredible son, Cree. I also dedicate it to you, the reader, whose life it may change.

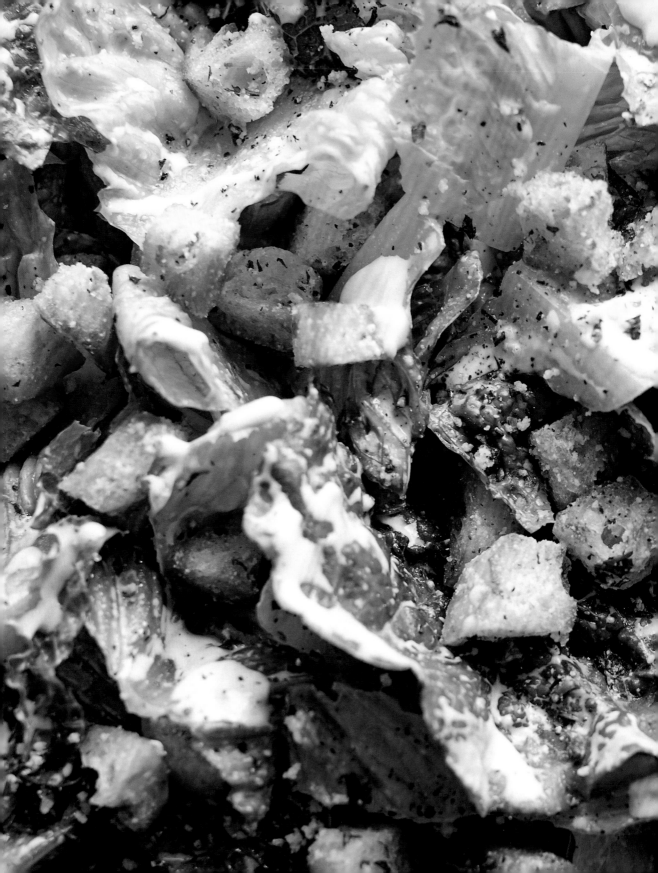

CONTENTS

Foreword

PERHAPS YOU PURCHASED TIA'S COOK-book because you've been a devoted fan for years; you want to know her beauty secrets and what fueled her rise to success at such an early age. How does she manage a busy, stressful life, yet seem so calm and composed? What is her secret to staying so fit? As an actress, a wife, and a busy mom, where does she find all that energy? What fuels her passionate determination to help those around her?

Well, this isn't just a cookbook. This is an honest, loving account of Tia's journey from an early childhood love affair with cooking delicious yet *harmful* foods to a new and healthier love affair with delicious yet *powerful* foods. Foods that actually heal.

From the very first page of *Whole New You*, you'll feel Tia's concern for *your* well-being. In spite of having been on television since her teen years, Tia has had life experiences very similar to your own. As a child, she was surrounded by junk food and didn't know that eating it would have serious consequences, such as lessening her chances of conceiving a child. The junk food led to bouts of illness for which Tia was given antibiotics that destroyed the colonies of beneficial microbes living in her intestines.

These microbes are one of the many wonders of the world: microscopic, invisible beings with huge power over us! They oversee and influence every function in the human body: manufacturing B vitamins that give us energy; helping us digest foods; balancing our hormones; and even controlling our thoughts, behaviors, and moods. Yes, right now the microbes in your gut are controlling your appetite and even your weight. Researchers now know that when certain species of microbes dominate the environment in the colon, they cause weight gain even if we are eating the healthiest foods.

Perhaps one of these microbes' most important functions is their influence on our immune system. Wipe them out with antibiotics, stress, or a high-fat, high-sugar diet and you wipe out your immune system. It literally loses control of your body, and tumors, pathogens, and opportunistic infections can take over. This is exactly what happened to Tia.

While it was exciting to star on a popular TV show, Tia was under constant pressure. Stress elevates the hormone cortisol, which then elevates blood sugar. Extra sugar in the blood, when it's there twenty-four hours a day, can cause a yeast infection that creates chronic inflammation (think of it as fire burning up your life force).

In Tia, this infection manifested as endometriosis: an overgrowth of tissue *outside* of the uterus that acts just like the tissue lining the *inside* of the uterus. The tissue eventually thickens and becomes inflamed, then breaks down and bleeds, but the blood can't flow out of the body. This can cause severe pain, scar tissue, and cysts and lead to infertility. Sadly, today millions of women suffer from endometriosis during their childbearing years. But there is hope: Through diet and lifestyle choices, Tia was able to turn this condition around and give birth to her son.

What Tia explains so clearly in this book is that food—deliciously enjoyable food—communicates with every cell in your body. It's a powerful tool and the secret to a more powerful *you*. Food is your foundation. Think about it: Right after you made the journey from your mother's womb to the outside world, what was the very first thing you did? You ate. Food is the basis for life. Real food—not the food most of us have eaten all our lives.

Food creates the energy you need to create the life you want. Food can correct faulty digestion. It can help to treat infections (such as candidiasis, herpes, and Lyme disease). Food can also help cleanse your body and allow it to protect you from the many dangerous environmental toxins that surround us today.

In *Whole New You*, Tia's bright, bubbly, kind, and wise spirit comes through loud and clear; she wants a better world for her son, for her family, and for us all. And she'd be the first to admit that her "spiritual self" is strengthened by the foods she now eats, which keep her centered.

So I congratulate you: Your own "spiritual self" compelled you to buy this book. But don't stop there! Schedule time on your calendar to make Tia's recipes. You will experience that same inner calm she feels in the kitchen and be filled with the energy that fuels her busy life. Not only is Tia sharing her favorite, absolutely delicious recipes with you, she's also taking you on an inspirational journey to discover who you really are.

For decades I've worked with men and women (mostly women) who have suffered from a myriad of health challenges. Everyone who has made the changes Tia recommends in this book has embarked on a healing journey. Finding the right foods for your unique body can improve, and often turn around, the most stubborn of health challenges.

This is the story of someone who healed herself, and who has all the happiness she ever dreamed possible. I witness many journeys to wellness in my work and I can tell you with certainty that nothing is more delicious than being healthy and fit and feeling great in your own skin.

    This isn't a diet book like the many on the market today. It's a treasure trove of inspiration, laughter, and powerful recipes that will change your life. Start to dine like Tia does and you won't be following a diet. You'll be learning how fantastic *real* food is.

Donna Gates

My Invitation to You

picked up *Whole New You*!

This book is an invitation—directly from me to you—to go on an adventure. It's not a Hollywood adventure; there won't be any pirates, or princesses, or bank heists. This adventure involves your body and your soul. It's a personal journey, and one that I've been on for a while now.

I want to help you see that food is powerful. And not only that: I want to help you see that *you* are powerful. By making some simple, easy choices, you can improve your life, and not just physically. By changing what you eat, you will experience emotional, mental, and even spiritual shifts.

I know because I've done it. I suffered from migraines my whole adult life. They're gone now. Eczema: Bye-bye! I even had endometriosis, a painful condition that makes it difficult and sometimes impossible to get pregnant. Now I look at my kid, who's going on five years old, and I marvel at him. I didn't overcome these challenges because I'm on TV, or because I live in Tinseltown, or because I'm somehow "special." I overcame them because I finally let go of denial and surrendered to the truth that what you eat *matters*. When I eat lousy food, I feel lousy. When I eat powerful food, I feel powerful. These are simple and humbling equations, for which I am extremely grateful.

We've all heard the saying "Food is medicine." But what does it really mean? I didn't understand it until, having exhausted all other paths to achieving good health, I *had* to begin thinking of food that way. It wasn't until I was doubled over in pain once again, until my doctor told me that I would find relief if I finally agreed to change my diet, that my mind opened to the concept.

You don't have to get to that place before seeking relief. I've written this book to help wake you up before a doctor has to shake you up. If you start experimenting now with the wonder of Nature's provisions, your path to healing can be an exciting and fun adventure, instead of a desperate measure propelled by a crisis.

You might already know all of this. Maybe you've been on your own journey for a while, and you're reading this over a green smoothie and a quinoa salad! If so, I hope that sharing my enthusiasm will bolster yours. Feel free to dive into the recipes for new ideas and tweaks on old classics—I look forward to seeing the delicious things you make when you share them with me on social media.

And if you're new to all of this, relax. I don't believe in big, heroic leaps. I know that life is messy, and that real change happens in teeny increments, and *never* according to anyone's timetable. I've suggested some little experiments you can try that will show you what food—and your body—are capable of. I've tried to explain things in ways that are fun and digestible. I've gone into some depth on the science, too—drawing many ideas from Donna Gates's *The Body Ecology Diet*, a cleansing, immune-boosting regimen that transformed my life—although we shouldn't need a study to tell us that broccoli is good for us (and can be super tasty roasted in the oven with a bit of lemon and olive oil).

Look: You're gonna have fantastic, mind-blowing insights . . . and, *perhaps,* some epic failures in the kitchen. Don't worry: I've almost burned down my house three times! I encourage you to maintain a sense of humor. There is no judgment here. I'm a busy mom with a crazy schedule and I don't even *aim* at perfection.

But I do aim at power. The power of Nature. The power of the body to heal itself. The power inside both you and me to make exciting, fantastic, life-changing choices.

You're officially invited to join me on this great adventure.

Are you in?

XO, Lia

WHOLE
NEW YOU

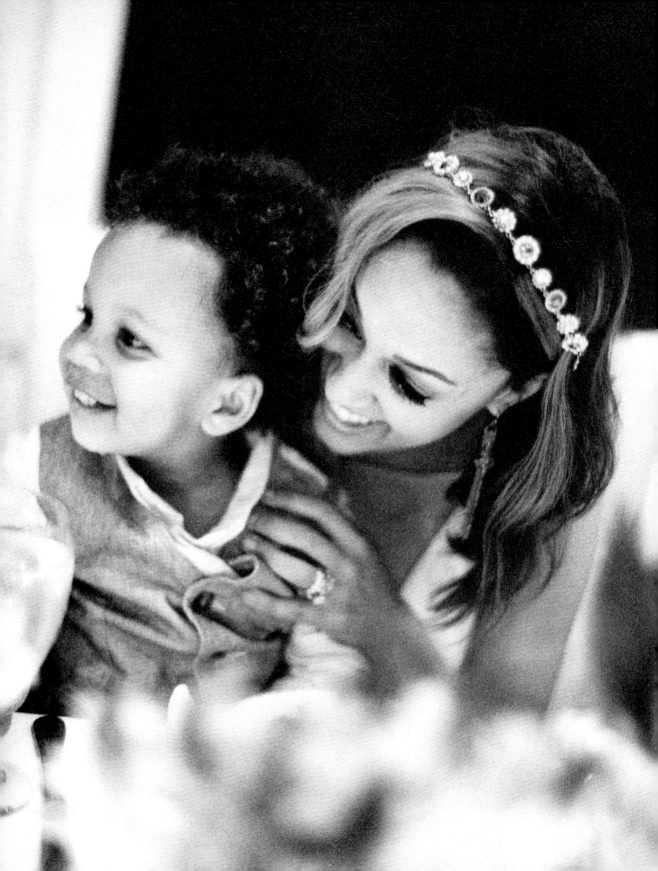

My Story

Kitchen Soldier

My mother loves to cook, and she, my grandmother, and all of my aunties can *throw down* some serious Southern classics. By the age of six, I was hanging out with them in the kitchen, and it was all about collard greens, mac 'n' cheese, chicken dishes—real soul food. I would watch and smell and taste as they performed their magic.

We were a military family—our mother was a drill sergeant and our father a first sergeant—so in our household, we all had chores. By the time I was twelve, I was cooking full meals for the family. By thirteen, I had mastered a variety of omelets, pork chops with mustard sauce, and even roasted Cornish hens. They weren't terribly fancy dishes, but having kitchen duty taught me basic cooking skills, patience, and an appreciation for home-cooked food.

In fact, I adored it. I would get absolutely *lost* in the kitchen. Because cooking had structure—bake this for fifteen minutes, add half a cup of that—I could relax within its boundaries. It was like a dance. To this day, I cook to relieve stress, sometimes to other people's amusement: When I fired up the stove on my last birthday, ready to start a quinoa dish, my husband, Cory, said, "Tia, you don't have to cook—it's your birthday! Why don't you just relax?" And I replied, while happily chopping a carrot, "Honey, you don't understand—this is my way of relaxing."

Have I mentioned that I love cooking?

Teen Extremes

My kitchen exploration stalled when my sister, Tamera, and I started shooting our TV sitcom, *Sister, Sister* at fourteen. Every morning, in the cafeteria at Paramount Studios, I would have a *stack* of pancakes. And when I say "stack" I mean at least four or five, topped with whipped cream, strawberries, and about a cup of maple syrup. And that was just breakfast.

TV sets are always catered, so I was surrounded by junk food, 24/7. To my teenage self, it was like living in Willy Wonka's chocolate factory. Everything I wanted was at my fingertips: Twizzlers, M&M's, Starbursts, potato chips, you name it. And if something I craved wasn't there, all I had to do was ask: "Chocolate chip cookies, please?" And they simply appeared. It was heaven.

If heaven leads to health problems, that is.

Nothing was fresh. Everything came out of a package, a bag, or a box. Every time I walked by the food table, I picked something up. And though I didn't know it at the time, an Oreo here and a bread roll there can lead to some nasty consequences.

I probably would have gained weight if, in my late teens, I hadn't started to use—and quickly abuse—diet pills. I didn't feel fat, but the pressure of being on television and wanting to look sexy and beautiful took over. I'm not proud of it. I got skinny, true, but the pills caused my heart to race, and I knew in my gut that I was hurting myself. A few years later, after the active ingredient in the pills was connected to a number of deaths, it got pulled from the market.

Around this time, I was also overusing antibiotics. No matter what symptom I presented to a doctor, even when all I had was the common cold, it seemed like I went home with antibiotics. This is really common. Don't get me wrong: Antibiotics are wonder drugs that have saved millions of lives. But they're doled out like aspirin. Antibiotics can zap a bacterial infection, but they also kill a lot of the *good* bacteria in the body, which is a big problem. (We'll get to that a little later. . . .)

In the last couple years of shooting *Sister, Sister,* I attended Pepperdine University part time. I was still eating lots of junk food and taking the diet pills, but I fell in love with student life. One of my favorite classes, Introduction to Psychology, was taught by a wonderful professor, Dr. Jeff Banks. He was fantastic. Everyone worshipped him because he seemed to understand our feelings and inner lives. His class wasn't just about grades; it was about *life*. Corny? Maybe. Meaningful? One hundred percent.

Part of the class was about unloading our own issues, fears, and troubles. I had never told anyone about the pills, but I got honest about them in class. Dr. Banks asked us to write down everything that we wanted to let go of and to make a promise to ourselves to address what was holding us back. I scribbled, "Give up diet pills" on a piece of paper, crumpled it up, and tossed it into the flames of my living room fireplace, just as Dr. Banks had instructed. As I watched the paper crackle and burn, something in me released. I haven't touched diet pills since that day, and thankfully, I haven't wanted to.

I did gain some weight, but I didn't care. By that point, my chest had started to hurt and I had discovered how dangerous the pills really were. I was grateful to be done with the speeding heart and the shame of having a secret. A few pounds were worth it.

La Dolce Vita

When *Sister, Sister* ended its six-year run, I was still in college, but comparatively speaking, I was free. I had more time, less responsibility, and university was opening my mind to totally new things. Up until that point, I'd always had the security of my parents and sharing a home with Tamera, and the structure of the TV show. Now something pushed me to get out of my comfort zone; I wanted to be challenged. So at twenty, I decided to go abroad.

I spent the summer in Italy, and took short trips from there to France, Spain, and Egypt. I was exposed for the first time to new languages, environments, and ways of life. I was stimulated on all levels and through all of my senses by the art, the architecture, and the smells on the streets. I had seen pictures of Michelangelo's *David* and the Florence Cathedral, but viewing them up close was another story. A new "me" blossomed. I may have spent my adolescence in front of an audience of millions, but I had been relatively sheltered. On this wonderful extended vacation, I visited the Vatican, sailed up the Nile, and drank my first glass of wine. I felt grown-up and sophisticated.

And the *food*. My taste buds were on fire! Goodbye, endless candy; hello, succulent chicken and frites in Paris, delicate thin-crust mushroom pizza in Florence (and, of course, gelato all over Italy), handmade bread in Cairo. There's nothing like it! Everything was made with quality ingredients and introduced me to tastes I'd never known. One of my most vivid memories is from Sardinia, where I was served a whole fish, on a beautiful platter, cooked to perfection. It was fresh, simple, and melted in my mouth.

Mmm . . .

Europe offered an almost orgasmic culinary experience, and it was there that my real love affair with food began. Until then, food and its preparation had represented a fun part of my childhood responsibilities and then the dangers of weight gain, but they had never been such artful and sensual *pleasures*.

The cook in me awakened. I asked myself, "What did they put in this?" and "How did they do *that*?" My inner twelve-year-old, who'd spent so much time in the kitchen, was back with a whole new set of tools and ingredients to explore. I couldn't wait to get home and start chopping.

Cory was my boyfriend at the time, and he picked me up at the airport after my trip. He could see immediately that I was a new person, inside and out. Not only had I awakened internally, I had gained fifteen pounds in two months, and he definitely approved: "Oh my god, Tia, *I love it!*" he said, as he slung my suitcase into the trunk of the car. I was round and juicy, with a big ol' booty. I felt fantastic.

But not for long.

Wake-Up Call

In 2006, I was still in college, and majoring in psychology. I was sitting in one of Dr. Banks's classes when I started to experience abdominal pain. It got so bad that I had to excuse myself. The only thing I could think to do was sit on the toilet, and that helped—a little. I missed the entire class, just sitting on the can. Tamera drove me home that day while I crouched in the backseat, doubled over.

A doctor did an ultrasound, which revealed a small ovarian cyst. She assured me that it would go away on its own, and that I would feel better soon. But I didn't. These painful episodes began to occur with regularity. During a particularly bad one, I followed all of the doctor's recommendations: I tried to relax, I took a hot bath, I placed a heating pad on my belly. Nothing worked and no one seemed to know how to help me. Baffled and terrified, I was *this close* to calling an ambulance. I knew, in my gut, that something was very, very wrong.

I decided to get a second opinion, and a friend recommended an ob-gyn named Dr. Kent, who had delivered Jada Pinkett Smith's babies. Dr. Kent also did an ultrasound and before she had even wiped the jelly off my belly, she declared, "I think you've got endometriosis."

I was confused. I'd never heard of endometriosis, although an estimated 15 percent of women get it; among African American women, the rate may be even higher. In those with the condition, the blood that's meant to build up every month on the *inside* of the uterus builds up on the outside instead. And that's a big problem. Not only does endometriosis cause incredible pain, it makes pregnancy pretty much impossible: If the uterine lining, where fertilized eggs implant and grow, is on the *outside* of the uterus, it's useless for baby-making.

It was scary to get the diagnosis, but a huge relief to receive an explanation for all the pain. Dr. Kent told me that the only way to confirm that I had endometriosis was to do surgery. By going inside, she could both diagnose and treat the condition. I hesitated; I'd never been under anesthesia, and I hated the idea of being poked and prodded.

"Do you want to have kids one day, Tia?" asked Dr. Kent.

I didn't have to think long or hard about that. "Yes," I said, "of course."

She looked at me in her kindly, doctorly way. "Then you should seriously consider surgery."

Bummer.

So I underwent laparoscopic surgery. After inserting a camera into my abdomen and assessing the situation, Dr. Kent told me, "You have endometriosis and several cysts." I wasn't too surprised by that, but what she said next threw me. "Tia," she said, "this is a chronic condition, and it will come back."

And it did. It took almost two years, but the symptoms finally returned. And when endometriosis comes back, it doesn't sneak in under the door; it comes *back*.

Tamera and I were out to lunch. We had just pitched a new series idea to a network executive. Over dessert, I was suddenly hit by a truckload of pain. Again, I was doubled over in agony, and again, poor Tamera had to help me home. I could see in her face that she felt helpless and afraid for me.

Dr. Kent put me on birth control pills, which can help with endometriosis, but after a while, she needed to put me on pain pills, too. After my nightmare with diet drugs, I had become pretty sensitive to what I put in my body, and I didn't like the idea of being dependent on pharmaceuticals. We talked about my options, and she recommended a second surgery. Cory and I were engaged at the time, and

I knew we were getting that much closer to planning for kids, so I agreed. I think, in that moment, part of me surrendered to having more and more surgeries as time went by. It was just what I had to do.

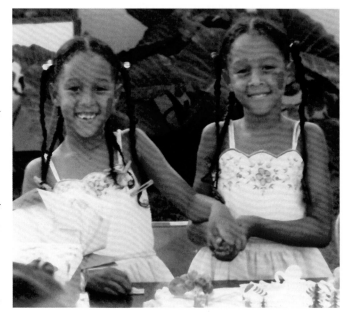

So, once again, I found myself on a cold operating table, under heavy anesthesia, and once again, Dr. Kent was using high-tech instruments and lasers to ease my suffering. It was like déjà vu. I came out of the surgery sore and saddened that this was going to be a recurring routine.

But this time Dr. Kent had another idea. At a checkup after my procedure, she sat me down, closed my file, and changed the course of my entire life: "If you want to stop having surgery, Tia . . ." she said, and then paused.

My heart leapt. I leaned in closer.

"If you want to get rid of your symptoms . . ."

This was getting good. Was there a new procedure? A permanent fix?

"If you want to have a baby . . ."

Oh God, yes, yes, YES!!! I thought. I'd do anything to have a baby. I sat poised for her solution, the medical knight in shining armor she was about to unleash.

"You have to change your diet, Tia."

I blinked.

And then I blinked again, not sure I'd heard her correctly.

"Especially dairy," she added, quite seriously. "You need to stop eating dairy. Now."

I was stunned.

It was the first time any doctor had connected my diet to my health. And to point a finger at dairy, no less? Wasn't dairy nature's perfect food? It made no sense.

"Your uterus is inflamed," she said. "And endometriosis is fueled by inflammation." That sort of made sense; blood on the outside of the uterus sounded . . . *inflamed*. Then she connected the big dots: "Dairy causes inflammation."

I looked at Dr. Kent, rocked by this new information. It had never even *occurred* to me that something I had always eaten (so innocently!) could be causing me such harm. Obviously, I'd heard the old adage "You are what you eat" a million times, but I'd never really processed that fundamental truth. Now here was a well-respected doctor telling me that my problem—my big, you-may-never-get-pregnant problem—came down to my favorite foods: butter, cheese, and gelato. It was like a slap in the face.

New Food, New Life

But I was equally stunned by the fact that I could do something about it. Dr. Kent sent me to a nutritionist, who confirmed that food and major health issues were definitely connected, and I kept on doing my own research. Then I reached out to a good friend, Brittany Daniel, my co-star on *The Game*, whom I'd worked with for five years. I knew that she had battled stage IV non-Hodgkins lymphoma, a very serious cancer—she's a rock star. In addition to going through chemotherapy, she had taken a particular approach to eating with amazing results, and she recommended I talk to Donna Gates, author of *The Body Ecology Diet*.

I met with Ms. Gates, who confirmed what Dr. Kent had said; not only was endometriosis fueled by inflammation, almost *all* diseases are supported by an inflamed condition in the body (we discuss this a little later). By fighting inflammation through diet, I could not only kick the endometriosis to the curb, I could prevent all sorts of other baddies!

I decided to go for it. Designed to reduce inflammation and strengthen the immune system, the Body Ecology diet meant letting go of all processed foods, refined sugar, and dairy. I also had to learn to cook with foods like quinoa and buckwheat that I'd never even *seen* before! A little meat was okay, but it had to be high quality—no antibiotics, no factory farms. I had to eat new vegetables—*lots* of them, and at every meal. This meant learning a new set of tricks in the kitchen. All told, it was a big shift.

Luckily, I'm a very determined woman, and when I want something, I get it. And I wanted to get pregnant very, very badly. So for a full year, while I was in Atlanta to shoot *The Game*, I followed the Body Ecology guidelines, with very few cheats. I was disciplined. Endometriosis had been like an alarm—a *loud* alarm—going off in my body, and I was finally ready to hear its message: Change how you eat!

Let's be real—I did it, but I wasn't *happy* about it. In fact, at first, it was extremely depressing. I didn't want to give up bread, cookies, noodles, and other refined carbohydrates. I felt like everything I loved was disappearing. I had devoted entire afternoons to watching *The Barefoot Contessa* and

Giada De Laurentiis, for crying out loud! My signature dish was cheesy pasta! When Cory's friends came around, I would make them deep-fried, breaded, cheese-filled tortellini!

You heard me. *Deep-fried.*

But now, my pasta and pizza days were gone. My trip to Italy, which had taught me to breathe from a deeper place, seemed like it had happened a thousand years ago. Food had been an orgasmic experience for me, and now?

Vegetables.

And unsurprisingly, I had to stay away from all processed foods, too: no chips, no Cheez Doodles, no pretzels. Nothing that came in a bag. Nothing from a package. Although I had dialed down my junk food consumption considerably since my trip to Europe, I hadn't cut it out altogether, and truth be told, I wasn't even sure if that was possible. (It was, of course; I had just never known that healthy food could be good for your body *and* good for your taste buds.)

Healthy foods carry a stigma that I'd like to erase. And it's not just because they've restored my health and turned my life around. It's not just because they're packed with nutrients and are simply good for you. I'm determined to push past that stigma because whole, natural foods, cooked with love, taste absolutely fantastic. You heard me: *fantastic.*

Okay, so I didn't feel that way overnight. But I persevered, and the benefits started rolling in: Within six months, the eczema I'd struggled with for years disappeared. My migraines evaporated. I lost weight, quickly and effortlessly. I was amazed.

As my body issues cleared up, my palate adjusted to all the new tastes I'd discovered, and I started to find natural foods delicious and truly *satisfying.* My food journey had come full circle: It began with the practical, as I learned to cook dinner for my family; it moved to the sensual, when I experienced a world beyond the one I had known; it became medicine when all else failed; and now it had begun to encompass all three.

As if that wasn't enough, I got a bigger surprise about a year after I began to eat this way: I started to feel deeply, thrillingly *alive.* I had more energy than I remembered ever having; my mind was clear and focused like a laser beam. For the first time in my life, I understood the concept of profound "wellness."

I started to do some research and learned that here in the West, we tend to concentrate on disease—focusing on the bits and pieces of the body and everything that can go *wrong* in its own discrete way. We get hypnotized by symptoms, and ignore their underlying causes. But in Chinese and many other traditional medicines, the doctor looks at the body as a whole, a system that is unified and self-healing. She focuses not on how to treat symptoms per se, but on how to support holistic wellness. By treating the whole body—and supporting it on all levels—many symptoms just disappear.

That's what was happening to me. By eating whole, natural, and clean food, I was supporting my body on a profound physical level. The food was detoxifying my blood, my organs, and my brain, changing everything. Like bodies do when they're treated right, mine was fixing itself. It was really cool.

I think you should feel that good, too. You deserve it. Are you ready?

Pregnancy

The cherry on top of this dairy-free sundae is that I got pregnant. Quickly. Given all my health issues, I hadn't expected it to happen so fast—if at all—but after I'd been following my new regimen for just twelve months, Cory came to visit me in Atlanta, and a few weeks later, we got the happy news!

I guess I'd just assumed that it would take longer, that the body couldn't repair itself *that* fast. We hadn't planned for pregnancy—it happened on the first try. But I was ecstatic; I wanted to start a family very badly. So I celebrated! With pizza. And ice cream. And Flamin' Hot *Cheetos*! (For weeks, I had the telltale orange fingers of the secret Cheetos-eater.)

I mean, I was pregnant, right? That was the whole point of the healthy eating stuff, no? I figured I didn't need to be so diligent anymore. Between my pregnancy-induced cravings and new laissez-faire attitude, my diet went all over the place.

Surprise! I paid for it. My migraines came back, worse than ever. My eczema returned. I had nosebleeds. But the worst issue was horrible, miserable nausea that lasted the duration of the pregnancy. Meanwhile, I was still shooting *The Game,* and my sister and I were doing our reality show, *Tia and Tamera*. I was throwing up so much that my doctor was considering putting me on an IV drip of Zofran, a heavy-duty anti-nausea drug.

I had heard that bread helped with nausea, so I ate bread. Loads and loads and *loads* of bread. It was the only thing I could keep down. I had no idea that, beyond causing weight gain, eating so much of one food could set me up for allergies and upset the balance of my body that I'd worked so hard to foster. I didn't know. I just ate more bread.

Sixty pounds later, I gave birth to Cree, our lovely baby son. That same day, the nausea simply went "Bye-bye!" After the pregnancy I was able to resume a more varied way of eating, but I didn't return to the Body Ecology principles . . . for a while.

Red Velvet Face

Soon after Cree's birth, Tamera and I were back on the set of *Tia and Tamera*. The show was doing really well, so to celebrate, Cory decided to surprise me with my favorite dessert: red velvet cupcakes. I indulged, and enjoyed them to the fullest.

But the next morning, during an interview at MTV, Tamera looked at me, horrified: "Tia!" she whispered, "Your *face!*" I had no idea what she was talking about until she adjusted her phone to show me my reflection; a big red rash was spreading over my whole face, and I looked like I'd aged thirty years. Needless to say, it was not a pretty sight.

An allergist diagnosed me with a yeast allergy. When I asked how it had happened, she told me,

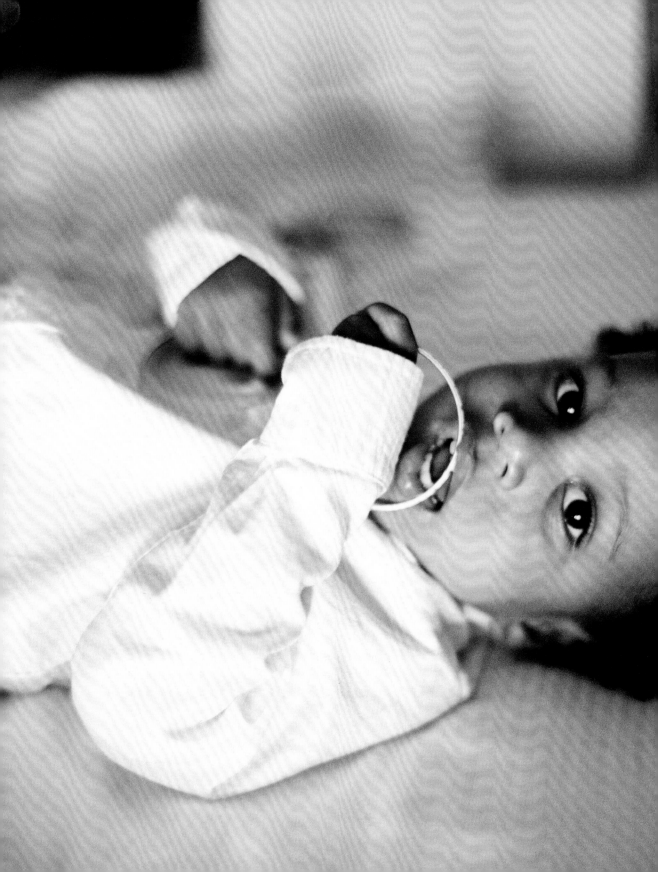

"The immune system can get imbalanced and sometimes it never gets back into balance." She explained that all the antibiotics I'd taken over the years had upset the balance of bacteria in my gut, which can affect the immune system. Not only that, she said, "You ate so much bread—and only *bread*—during most of your pregnancy. That can lead to an allergy." And all it took was a yummy little cupcake to set it off.

Red Velvet Face was a final wake-up call for me. There was no turning my back on the truth that my body was profoundly affected by what I put in my mouth, no matter how gooey and delicious. That cupcake notified me—in a pretty gross way—that, like many people, I suffer from an overgrowth of Candida albicans, a natural yeast in the body. I returned to an extra-clean diet to get myself back in balance. Since then, I have happily settled into eating foods that work for me: clean, powerful, whole foods.

Which doesn't mean I do it perfectly. I have my ups and downs, my backs and forths. But every time I eat something processed, or highly refined, or just plain over the top, I feel it. Not in a horrible truckload-of-pain-endometriosis way, thank God. Now it's just little alarm bells, ringing from deep down inside: "Tia . . . Tiiiiiiaaaaaa!!!"

How to Use This Book

I WROTE THIS BOOK BECAUSE EATING SUPER HEALTHY FOOD HEALED my body, improved my life, and helped me have a baby. But in order to recover from endometriosis, I had to stick to a pretty strict regimen, for over a year. For the body to really clean itself—from the inside out—it needs simple, balanced food for a sustained period of time. I was really motivated to be strict because I was severely out of balance; I was in pain, and needed change.

But I should say, before we get started, that this book is not designed to address diagnosed or specific medical conditions; although I've had my own powerful healing experience, that does not give me the expertise or the credentials to offer specific healing advice to anyone with a serious condition. This book is for my friends, family, and fans; I've written it so you can feel utterly amazing, look gorgeous, and avoid serious problems down the road. Because *Whole New You* suggests that you give up dairy, white sugar, and processed foods—while gorging on vegetables, whole grains, and other healthy delights—absorbing its messages will be a profound and positive experience, especially if you're currently on the Standard American Diet. And it will spur you to make other moves in the direction of health. The *Whole New You* way of eating will change your life.

For those of you who are currently wrestling with a serious health problem, it's important that you seek out medical guidance while learning to support yourself with a healthier diet. If you're interested in exploring a deep internal overhaul, I recommend you read *The Body Ecology Diet*. Every condition is different, and that book goes deeper into the details of a comprehensive detox, like the one I did.

And to make things clear for every type of reader, I've given the recipes little labels, so you know what you're getting:

Dishes I ate during my healing diet are marked: CLEAN

clean

Recipes that I make less often or on special occasions, like chocolate cake or fried chicken, are marked: FUN

fun

Recipes that are 100 percent plant-based recipes are marked: VEGAN

veg

And finally, gluten-free recipes are marked: GLUTEN-FREE

g-f

Beyond being healthy, the one thing that all the recipes have in common? They are 100 percent delicious.

I can't wait for you to try them!

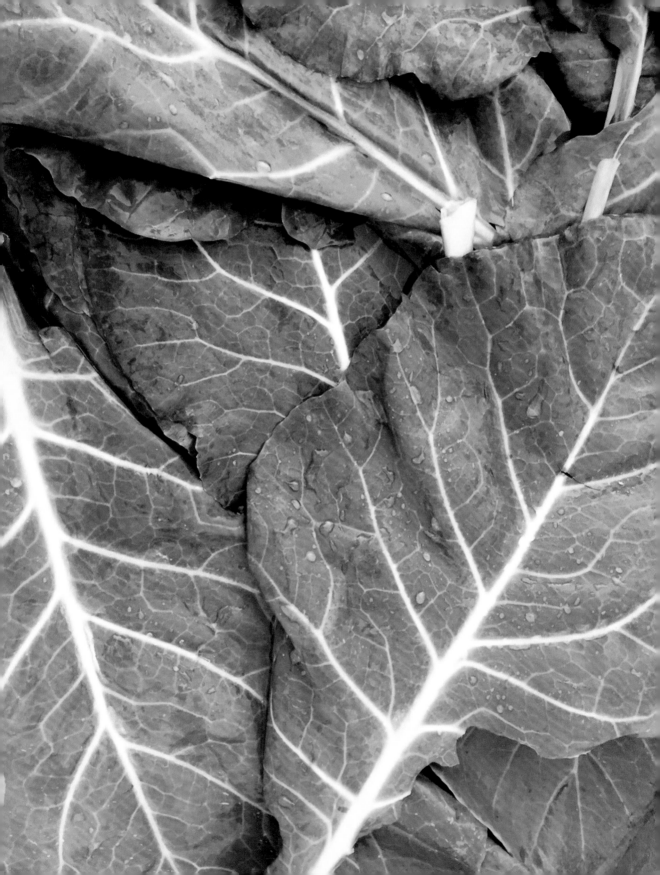

Three Big Concepts

WHEN I WAS DIAGNOSED WITH ENDOME-
triosis, my whole perspective shifted. Not only
was I confronted with a serious health condition,
my doctor actually encouraged me to take some
responsibility for it. It was as if she gently held up
a mirror and said, "You played a role in this, Tia."

Obviously, I hadn't done it consciously—no
normal person would seek out the pain that was
battering my belly. But I had done it uncon-
sciously, through a series of little choices that
had pushed my body in the wrong direction. On
my healing journey, I learned a lot about how to
approach health and nutrition. But three big concepts stood out, and I've written this book to
share them with you because they apply to us all.
I hope they'll make you feel as empowered as I
did when I first learned them.

You Are Whole, and
Your Body Works Perfectly

From the outside, it's easy to perceive the body as a bunch of individual pieces: Here are my hands, there's my head, and these are my boobs. Western medicine encourages this compartmentalization, and we have doctors who specialize in different bits and pieces.

But on the *inside*, everything is connected. Think about it: The air you breathe goes to every cell, without prejudice. The blood in your arteries circulates from the top of your head to the tips of your toes, and then repeats its loop again and again and again. The food you eat nourishes your bones and your biceps and your butt alike. From the *inside*, you are a symphony of fluid, tissue, and organs, all working together to keep this amazing miracle of a body playing its personal song.

Which is pretty cool.

And it gets even cooler: As you read this—right at this very moment—more than 30 *trillion* cells, each with your personal DNA signature, are chugging away, every one carrying out its specific, microscopic job—just for you—in perfect harmony with all the others. They are separate, and yet they share an intelligence that helps them behave as a whole. At any given moment, millions are being born, and millions are retiring. These cells are in motion while you read, while you work, and even while you sleep.

Right now, your body is handling your temperature, your respiration, and your heartbeat. It's growing your hair, your nails, and new layers of skin. Its delicate system of glands is whispering hormonal instructions through your bloodstream like "Grow tissue," "Get aroused," and "Menstruate." If you've ever been pregnant, you are familiar with the hormonal fireworks displays your body is capable of!

And underneath all this activity, your body's primary mission is to keep you healthy; that's its thing, its *obsession*. It does absolutely everything, from recoiling from a hot flame to carrying out a circus of chemical reactions, in order to maintain one single thing: your health.[*]

Meanwhile, we sit around obsessing about our thigh dimples.

So being healthy isn't so much about following the perfect set of rules; it's not about making a Herculean effort to achieve some beyond-your-reach state of "fitness." Your body is *fine*. It's more than fine, in fact. Your miraculous body knows exactly what to do—on several different levels of mind-numbing complexity—better than you, or I, or even science will ever understand. It's doing them all right now!

---

[*] Of course, some of us are born with differently abled bodies. Even so, the body is designed to do everything it can to thrive, in spite of serious impediments. This isn't about being a superhero—it's about being the best **you** you can be.

Your job . . . is to get out of its way.

And that's what my doctor was basically saying to me that day: "Tia, get out of your body's way. Just stop *hurting* it." She knew that my body wanted nothing more than to heal itself, and was entirely capable of doing it. The only thing it needed was my cooperation.

In this respect, my MD was practicing more holistically, like an acupuncturist would. As I mentioned before, Eastern medicine understands the body as a whole, constantly seeking health and balance. The practitioner's job is to support the entire system by releasing stuck energy and gently stimulating points of weakness. To an acupuncturist, the idea of focusing exclusively on one organ—or any single body part—would be absurd, since everything is connected. The whole affects the part, and the part affects the whole. A practitioner of Chinese medicine uses natural herbs, dietary recommendations, and needles the width of a single hair to gently coax the body back into balance.

But we are getting ahead of ourselves.

All you need to do right now is to begin thinking about your body differently, with more respect for your wholeness and its wisdom. Looking at yourself through this lens, you are no longer just your hair, or your fingernails, or even your thigh dimples!

CONCEPT #2:

Inflammation Is a Thing

Your body's mission is to keep you healthy. And I don't just mean in a behind-the-scenes way. You are likely already familiar with your body's more obvious displays of its badass healing superpowers. For instance: When you bang your forehead on the cabinet, it starts to swell up within seconds. You get a bump, it turns red, and it even gives off heat, in a nifty little healing process that neutralizes harmful microorganisms and repairs your wound. This is called inflammation, and it's your immune system in action: a fantastic response to life's mishaps. So inflammation is awesome—even life-saving—when it's necessary. Thank goodness for inflammation!

The word "inflammation" comes from the Latin "inflammatio," which means fire!
IS IT GETTING WARM IN HERE?

But that's only half the story. In our modern age, we are seeing a different type of inflammation. Instead of the body responding to acute problems, like a whack on the head, many people are experiencing chronic inflammation—a sort of low-level inflammation—*all the time*. Our immune systems are flaring up when they don't need to.

Think of it this way: If you have chronic inflammation, your body is acting like a burner that's turned on, day and night. Instead of being nice and cool most of the time and heating up only when you need it to, your body is on a constant low simmer. And because the body is not designed to simmer all the time, the condition eventually causes damage, weakness, and finally a breakdown. You burn out, so to speak.

Except you don't feel it. It's a *quiet* inflammation, and it can go on for years without detection until a symptom arises. And even then, most doctors will treat the symptom without addressing how the underlying inflammation started in the first place.

This kind of inflammation can show up in many ways: Arthritis (inflamed joints), colitis (inflamed colon), and sinusitis (inflamed sinuses) are just three of the conditions that end in "-itis," which means . . . drumroll . . . *inflammation*. But it doesn't stop with the "itises"; my endometriosis was driven by inflammation, and big baddies like heart disease, diabetes, and even cancer are all linked, quite directly, to chronic inflammation.

So what causes inflammation? Well, we've determined that the body uses it to fix things that are going wrong; it's the body's response to damage or to a foreign invader that wants to make us sick. *Chronic* inflammation occurs when there is *continual* damage being done to tissue, or when pathogens are being let in too easily and often. Stress and environmental toxins can be triggers. But ultimately, it's really the crappy food we put in our bodies—three times a day, 365 days a year—that may be doing the greatest damage. Modern food contains highly refined sugar, unnaturally processed vegetable oils, chemical stabilizers, dyes, and other non-foodstuffs. These ingredients cause the body's immune system to freak out in its attempt to repair all the damage that they do.

And it's not just processed foods. As my doctor told me, even dairy causes inflammation. Think about it: It's the mother's milk of another species, full of hormones and potent compounds designed for a baby cow—and even *cows* stop drinking it after infancy. Doesn't it make sense that the human immune system might get pushed into high alert by another species' DNA and start asking, "What is *this*?"

Poor immune system. And it gets worse: When the immune system is activated all the time, *it* ends up doing damage as well. It doesn't mean to, but it's not supposed to be turned to "ON" all the time! It can't keep on working at high intensity all day, every day, without something going wrong.

And that's on us.

In this book, you will be learning how to choose and cook foods that are anti-inflammatory. But what that really means is that they're natural. Guess what? Foods that Nature creates for humans *don't alarm the immune system*. Imagine that! And the less processed a food, the less inflammation it causes. If you're currently in good health, it's probably okay to ingest some weird stuff every once in a while, but eating foods that cause inflammation all the time is dumb, and will eventually become dangerous.

Take it from me.

CONCEPT #3:

You Are Not Alone

It's very difficult to achieve anything sustainable without a support system. We all work within systems—at home, at work, within our communities—to get things done. A TV show wouldn't make it to air without a crew, the president couldn't run this country without a staff of hundreds, and where would Santa be without his elves? Think of all the helpers in your life—family, friends, co-workers, teachers, religious or spiritual guides, even the farmers who grow your food and the waste management people who pick up your trash. All of these people work in a silent symphony to help you live your life.

It's an amazing system.

Well, you have helpers on the *inside* of your body, too. Get this: You have microscopic bacteria in you—and on you—that are constantly helping you to stay healthy. I know, it sounds a little gross—but bear with me.

There's no getting around it. We have evolved *in tandem* with these bacteria. So before you go and drink a bottle of hand sanitizer, understand that not only are these bacteria good, they are absolutely essential to your well-being. In the last decade, doctors and scientists all over the world have been waking up to these critters and the role they play in human health. There is a resounding consensus that our inner bacteria, or "microbiome," may be the key to our whole immune system.

Step away from the Purell.

Understand that you will never see or feel these microbes because they are so incredibly tiny. So tiny, in fact, that you carry 100 trillion bacterial cells in your small intestine alone. That's more bacterial cells than human cells, just in your gut!

And they work hard for you, helping to break down your food and digest it properly. Without them, foods don't get assimilated well, which leads to all sorts of problems, such as food allergies and even what's called "leaky gut," which is when minuscule holes are created in the small intestine. Leaky gut is really serious, because all the stuff that should have been stopped by your friendly bacteria—bad bacteria, toxins, indigestible foods, and even viruses—moves into your undefended bloodstream and wreaks all sorts of havoc. Individuals suffering from chronic diarrhea, brain fog, memory loss, or excessive fatigue might do well to learn about the microbiome and how they can help it thrive.

Happily, new research is suggesting that *healthy* gut bacteria produce neurotransmitters like dopamine (the pleasure chemical), serotonin (the mood stabilizer), and GABA (which calms us down) and can have a direct and positive impact on our brains, behavior, and mental health. A healthy party in your gut means a healthy party in your brain.

And there's more: It is now believed that up to 75 percent of your immune system function occurs in your gut. You see, you have a mix of friendly and nasty bacteria in your small intestine, but the good guys generally beat the bad. They are your first line of defense against microbial invaders. Friendly bacteria are constantly killing unfriendly bacteria, keeping them at bay.

Little ninja dudes.

And when these badass critters are doing their job, your immune system doesn't have to be putting out fires constantly, and that means—remember Concept #2?—less inflammation. Hooray! Also, when these good bacteria *do* detect a problem, they activate a set of immune system responses so that your body can go into full-fight mode. It seems the microbiome of the gut has its own unique intelligence.

However, the microbiome is extremely complicated, involving many types of bacteria and our equally complicated immune system . . . and this is where my lack of a science or medical degree brings us to a thudding halt. Not only are the details too nuanced to explain in this book, but more information is being discovered as I write; this field of science is new and exciting.

But it turns out we don't need to fully understand our gut bacteria in order to influence them, in both good and bad ways. We know now that antibiotics—although miraculous when fighting serious infections—take a big toll, effectively wiping out many of your friendly critters every time you pop a pill. So when antibiotics are over-prescribed, like they were for me, they weaken the immune system—in my case, leading to Candida overgrowth.

> **WHAT IS CANDIDA?** Candida albicans is a naturally occurring yeast in the human body—we all have it—which is normally kept in check by friendly bacteria in the gut. When gut bacteria become depleted or imbalanced, Candida can get out of control and take over the gut, where it begins to wreak havoc: Hello, bloating, fatigue, foggy brain, and a host of other symptoms. Unchecked, Candida can spread to the throat, nails, vagina, butt, and skin. At its very worst, it can travel through the entire body, causing fungal infections, autoimmune diseases, and skin issues. NO FUN!

And I didn't get antibiotics just from the pharmacy. Cattle and other livestock raised on factory farms or through other big industrial operations are regularly dosed with antibiotics to not only prevent infection, but to bulk the animals up. By eating that meat, I was getting a secondary load of antibiotics, weakening my gut flora even more.

The good news is that you can restore your gut's health easily! By eating naturally fermented, cultured vegetables (see page 211), unpasteurized pickles, and traditionally fermented foods like miso, you will begin to feed your small intestine good-quality bacteria. Just like you can build your muscles by going to the gym, you can boost your microscopic buddies when your immune system is out of whack. It's simple and delicious. You don't need a medical degree to support your own health.

Just a head of cabbage.

———

So that's it. Three big concepts: You are whole; inflammation is a thing; and you are not alone. Each is a new way of looking at yourself, your body, and how you can live a healthier, happier life.

So now we are ready to talk about food. Mmm . . . *food*.

In the next chapter, we are going to look at two types of foods—those that heal and those that hurt—and examine each through the lens of the Three Concepts, asking:

1. *Is it whole?*
2. *Does it cause inflammation?*
3. *Is it good for your gut bacteria?*

Let's get started!

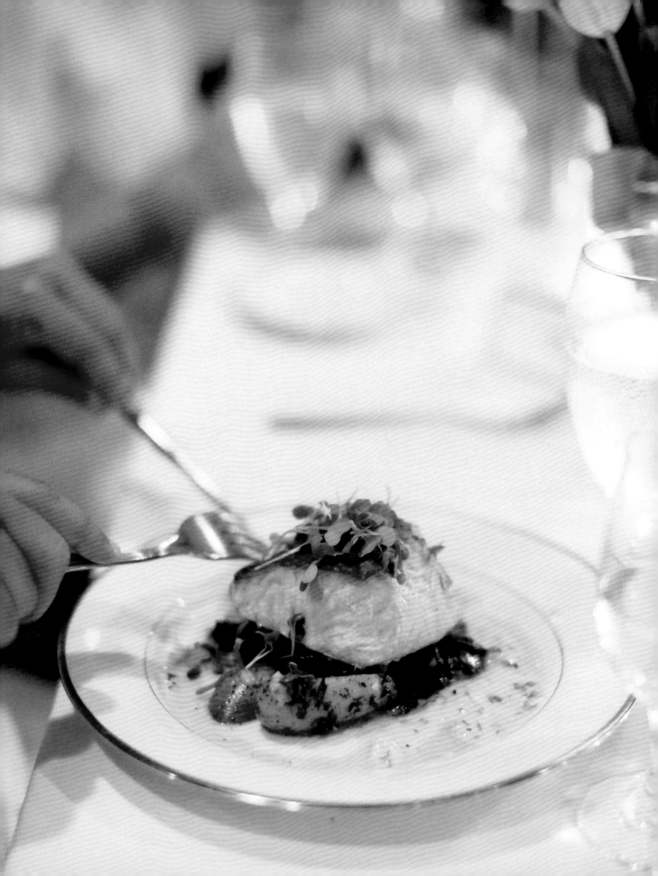

The Power of Food

FOOD IS POWERFUL AND HAS A SIGNIFicant impact. No matter what you put in your mouth—the good, the bad, or the Cheeto—it's doing *something*.

We are encouraged to think of food as simply fuel, but it's so much more than that. Every time you eat, you are building your *life*—creating your next moment, your next mood, and even your future successes. Your choices matter!

But no one's perfect; I still make less-than-stellar choices every once in a while. That's life. However, I've done the (sometimes painful) research and learned which foods support me best, and I choose the ones that work for me *most of the time*. That's experience.

This chapter is dense. It gets into the nittygritty. You will learn about both the foods that help and those that hurt . . . and why. It's interesting stuff, but you don't have to read this chapter before diving into the recipes themselves. In fact, please make a yummy snack to nosh on while you read. Remember, the food has actual power, so *eating* it is much more important than *understanding* it. This chapter is designed to illuminate, inspire, and educate, but it's your fork that'll do the heavy lifting.

So read a little and eat a little. Read some more and eat some more. Chew on the food as you chew on the information. This process is deep and real and will continue for the rest of your life, so relax and enjoy.

THE GOOD NEWS: *Foods that Heal*

FIRST, WE ARE GOING TO AIM AT THE GOOD FOODS: THE ONES WE ARE INVITING into our lives, with open arms! Some of them may seem new to you—or even sound a little weird—but trust me, they have become my best friends and I'm sure you will learn to love them, too.

They are:

- Whole Plant Foods
- High-Quality Protein
- Sea Vegetables
- Fermented Foods
- Safer Sweets

And, like I said before, we are going to look at each food through the lens of the Three Concepts, asking:

1. *Is it whole?*
2. *Does it cause inflammation?*
3. *Is it good for your gut bacteria?*

The answers to those questions will give us lots of juicy information, so let's get started:

Whole Plant Foods

By whole plant foods, I mean vegetables, whole grains, fruits, nuts, and seeds—all in their natural form. This doesn't mean you can never cut them up or take off their skins, but you should be buying them fresh (or dried, for grains and seeds), and rarely from a box or a bag. Let's consider whole plant foods using the Three Concepts.

1. *Are they whole?*

Absolutely. You may not eat every bit of them, but they're still whole. And this *wholeness* is really important.

Remember when we talked about your body being whole and working perfectly? Well, Nature gives us foods in their whole forms, too. And it's in this form that most foods work the best for our health. Whole plant foods contain lots of good things: complex carbohydrates, fiber, vitamins, and minerals—we all know that—but what nutrition scientists are just discovering is that these elements work best in *conjunction* with each other; they have synergy.

For instance, the natural sugar in a grain of brown rice hits your bloodstream very slowly and peacefully because the fiber in the grain slows it down. What a cool system! If the fiber is absent—that is, if the bran has been removed—the grain's sugar is absorbed too quickly, which causes tons of problems (we'll talk more about that in the "Sugar and Other Highly Refined Carbohydrates" section on page 47).

Another example is kale: The iron in kale is absorbed into your body very efficiently because it also contains lots of vitamin C. Without the vitamin C, not much of the iron would get into your body in a usable form. Go kale!

Nature isn't dumb. We need to realize that it has created a perfect delivery system for every food, one that we're only just beginning to understand. We spent the last seventy years thinking that we could outwit Nature, "improving" and "refining" and "enriching" foods, but guess what? We've been making ourselves sick! And all the while, the answer has been waiting in a grain of brown rice, as it whispers, *"Eat me!"*

2. *Do whole plant foods cause inflammation?*

No. Just the opposite.

In general, whole plant foods are anti-inflammatory—especially vegetables, which tend to alkalize the body. You can never go wrong eating tons and tons of veggies. Most grains, fruits, nuts, and seeds are slightly acidic (compared to vegetables), but they have strong anti-inflammatory properties, too. For example, all whole plant foods contain powerful antioxidants that actively smack down inflammatory compounds known as *free radicals*. Plants are your personal bodyguards.

Which is pretty awesome, you must admit.

Of course, as soon as plant foods get processed—refined, with additives, preservatives, or unnatural flavors—they have a different impact, and can cause any number of imbalances. Remember: *Wholeness* is the key.

3. *Are whole plant foods good for gut bacteria?*

Hell yeah.

Your friendly bacteria LOVE these foods. Remember, your microscopic helpers have evolved alongside the human race, and that means they were hanging around in the guts of your ancestors, and *their* cavemen ancestors, and whoever was here before that. These guys are *old*. They love whole foods because that's what they've eaten for thousands of years.

Here's a list of some of the foods we are discussing. Such amazing abundance!!!

VEGETABLES

Beets
Bok Choy
Broccoli
Burdock
Cabbage
Carrots
Cauliflower
Celery
Chard
Collard Greens
Kale (Curly, Red
    Russian, and
    Lacinato)
Leeks

Lettuce
Mushrooms
    (technically a
    fungus, but
    we consider
    it a veg)
Mustard Greens
Napa Cabbage
    (or Chinese
    Cabbage)
Onions
Parsnips
Peppers
Potatoes

Radishes (including
    Chinese Radish,
    Daikon)
Romanesco
Rutabaga
Spinach
Summer Squash
Tomatoes
    (technically a
    fruit, but hey)
Turnip Greens
Turnips
Winter Squash
Zucchini

WHOLE GRAINS

Amaranth
Brown Basmati Rice
Brown Rice
Buckwheat
Farro

Kamut
Millet
Quinoa
Rye
Spelt

Teff
Whole Barley
Whole Oats
Whole Wheat Berries
Wild Rice

FRUITS

Apples
Apricots
Bananas
Berries
Coconuts
Dates
Figs

Grapefruits
Kiwis
Lemons
Mangoes
Melons
Oranges
Papayas

Peaches
Pears
Persimmons
Pineapples
Plums
Pomegranates

NUTS

Almonds	Hazelnuts	Pecans
Brazil Nuts	Macadamia Nuts	Pistachios
Cashews	Peanuts	Walnuts

SEEDS

Chia	Poppy	Sunflower
Flax	Pumpkin	
Hemp	Sesame	

DO I NEED TO BUY ORGANIC PRODUCE? If you can afford to get 100 percent organic foods, that's great. Organic fruits and vegetables generally taste better, and a recent review of over 300 studies showed that organic produce did contain more nutrients than conventionally grown produce.[1] Grains and beans are pretty cheap, no matter what, so the organic versions shouldn't break your bank.

That said, I don't want you to get all neurotic about this stuff. The most important thing is that you eat more vegetables and other whole plant foods, organic or not! And if you can buy only *some* organic fruits and veggies, try to pick from the following list—these are foods that are sprayed with the most pesticides, so it's best to get them organic:

THE FOLLOWING FOODS ARE SPRAYED WITH THE MOST PESTICIDES

- Apples
- Blueberries (domestic)
- Celery
- Cherry Tomatoes
- Cucumbers
- Grapes
- Hot Peppers
- Nectarines (imported)
- Peaches
- Potatoes
- Snap Peas (imported)
- Spinach, Kale, and Collards
- Strawberries
- Sweet Bell Peppers

Meanwhile, there's another group of foods that absorb very little pesticide, so you don't need to buy their organic variety unless you want to. They are:

- Asparagus
- Avocados
- Cabbage
- Cantaloupe
- Eggplants
- Grapefruits
- Kiwi Fruits
- Mangoes
- Onions
- Pineapples
- Sweet Corn (although I prefer organic corn, because it's not genetically modified)
- Sweet Peas
- Sweet Potatoes
- Watermelon

WHAT ABOUT FLOUR? You might assume that whole-grain noodles and whole-grain breads are whole foods. I mean, they still contain all their bits and pieces, right? Well, yes and no. Although whole-grain bread does contain fiber, complex carbs, and the original nutrients from the grain, it doesn't actually count as a whole grain, per se, because it no longer has its original energy. A whole grain (like a grain of brown rice, or a whole wheat berry) contains all its vital bits and pieces, intact and in their natural relationships to one another. This allows the grain to maintain its vital force of "chi"* that diminishes considerably when that same grain is ground into a flour—and your body knows it. Try this experiment: cook up a pot of brown rice, whole barley, or whole wheat berries (see the chart on page 199). Serve yourself a scoop, chew it really well, and notice the energy that fills you. Groove on that for a bit. Then eat a piece of bread and observe its effect on your body. Flour tends to be harder to digest and can have a sludgy effect on the body's energy.

Fear not: I'm not here to steal away all your sandwiches and pasta dishes. Whole-grain flour products can be a lovely part of a healthy and delicious life. But please don't get them confused with actual whole grains, which contain powerful energy, and should be prioritized in your diet.

---

* Also known as *ki*, *qi*, or *prana*, this invisible life force is recognized in all major Eastern healing traditions, dating back thousands of years. It's the force underlying *our* wholeness, and the one that acupuncturists and holistic healers seek to strengthen and support when a patient is sick.

More Good News about
Whole Plant Foods

WHOLE PLANT FOODS GIVE YOU ENERGY: All whole plant foods contain lots and lots of carbohydrates.

Wait. Aren't we supposed to run away—screaming—from carbs?

Not at all. You see, we've gotten confused about carbs. Carbohydrates are not only good, they are absolutely essential to the human body. Carbohydrates provide the glucose that your cells use to make energy. Without carbs, you'd have no gas in your tank.

However, just like at the gas station, you have a choice in the quality of fuel you buy: You can get your fuel from *simple* carbohydrates or *complex* carbohydrates. Simple carbs (like white sugar, white flour, and fruit juices) go straight to your bloodstream. Think of them as FAST carbs. If you're falling into a diabetic coma, you want a fast carb to jerk you out of it, but in everyday life, they can wreak havoc.

Complex carbohydrates are the SLOW carbs. Whole grains, vegetables, nuts, and seeds are all rich in these complex carbs. They break down slowly, allowing your body to use them efficiently—over a few hours—and the energy they create is beautiful. Slow carbs make you feel steady, coordinated, and able to meet all of life's challenges. Your brain loves these carbs, as they make for clear and happy thinking. You will write symphonies, poems, and world-saving computer code on slow carbs!

CHEWING: The more you chew complex carbs—veggies, whole grains, and even whole-grain flour products—the sweeter they get. That's because thorough chewing actually breaks down the sugars in your mouth, using a special enzyme in your saliva called amylase. And the more sugar you release from the food, the more energy you feel! Yes, even if you don't chew, these foods will eventually be digested in your small intestine, but not as efficiently, and you won't get the same satisfaction or energy from them. News flash: You have molars, and saliva, *for a reason*!

I'm not great at doing it, but when I practice some championship chewing—chewing thirty to fifty times per mouthful—I feel amazing. Try it.

WHOLE PLANT FOODS MAKE YOU LIVE LONGER: In his book *The Blue Zones: 9 Lessons for Living Longer from the People Who've Lived the Longest,* Dan Buettner researched the cultures of people who live the longest on the planet. These included the Japanese living on the island of Okinawa, the people of Sardinia, and members of the Seventh-Day Adventist Church living in Loma Linda, California. Among a number of factors that favored longevity, a diet *rich in complex carbohydrates* ranked among the highest. A recent meta-study conducted at Harvard found that people who ate whole grains on a regular basis lived longer and healthier lives than those who didn't.[2] Whole foods aren't just for hippies!

WHOLE PLANTS HAVE FIBER: Whole plant foods have insane amounts of fiber. And fiber, even though it sounds like something your granny would stir into her coffee at breakfast, is cool. Think of fiber as the bulky part of any plant food, the scaffolding around which the other nutrients organize themselves. The strings in celery? The veins in a collard leaf? The bran of a whole grain? All fiber.

Fiber:

- Lowers cholesterol
- Slows down the absorption of carbs
- Balances and helps to discharge excess hormones
- Sweeps toxins out of your body
- Makes you feel full
- Makes great poops
- Is one of your bacterial critters' favorite foods

Fiber isn't just for grandma. Maybe grandmas talk about fiber so much because they know what's up!

GLUTEN

Gluten-free foods are all over the place these days. Every celebrity, friend-of-a-friend, and co-worker has declared herself "gluten-intolerant." But what's the real deal with gluten?

Gluten is a protein that shows up in wheat, barley, and a few other grains. If you've ever kneaded a ball of dough and felt it get spongy and expansive, you've activated its gluten. Gluten gives baked products their elasticity and resilience.

Baguette, anyone?

However, some people react to gluten as a foreign invader, and for them it provokes a strong inflammatory reaction. For people with celiac disease, gluten is utterly indigestible and produces serious damage to the gut, making almost *all* foods indigestible.

Ugh. It's *bad*.

If you suspect you have problems with gluten, you may want to get a simple blood test that will tell you if you have celiac disease, which is genetic.

If you suspect you have a gluten sensitivity, you might (it's becoming more common, with our Western diets, and related to our immune system issues), but you also might be reacting to refined flour. Milled into a paste, lacking fiber and other nutrients, flour can be difficult to digest and can leave the eater feeling bloated, gassy, and unsatisfied. These sensations are attributed to gluten, but they may be triggered by the refined foods you're eating.

Try this test: Soak and cook organic, whole wheat berries (the whole grains, with their fiber intact, which you can find in bulk at health-food stores; see the chart on page 199) and see how you feel after eating them. Wheat contains gluten, but the gluten you're getting from the berries isn't in the form of sticky, broken-down flour. If you still feel discomfort and want to stay away from gluten altogether, more power to you. If you don't, you may just want to reduce your flour intake and, when you do eat flour products, chew them very thoroughly, which will help enormously in digesting them.

I've marked all the recipes in this book that contain gluten so you can modify them according to preference.

WHOLE PLANT FOODS CONTAIN PHYTONUTRIENTS: Nutrition scientists are only just beginning to figure out exactly what vegetables and other whole plant foods can do. They've known for a long time that veggies and grains have vitamins, minerals, and fiber. But recently, they've discovered the presence of "phytochemicals"—meaning *plant* chemicals—that are truly amazing.

Here are just three of them:

- Carotenoids give vegetables their bright colors, and scientists have identified more than six hundred so far. Carotenoids clean up the damage done to cells by pollution, other toxins, and radiation. Plus, they improve your immune function. Not bad.
- Lignans come from plant cell walls, and basically regulate your hormones. Thank you, lignans!
- Glucosinolates are found in cruciferous vegetables, and they . . . get this: prevent certain *cancers*. Nice job!

MEDICINE IS FOOD: I know, I've been like a broken record telling you that food is medicine. But did you know that most medicines are derived from foods? Plants, to be exact. That's because plants are so powerful. Yes, modern medicine has refined, rejiggered, and concentrated certain plant compounds to make them even more potent, but their original medicinal properties were discovered in jungles, fields, and forests! For example, aspirin comes from the willow plant, many heart medicines come from the foxglove plant, and even a treatment for ovarian cancer, called Taxol, is derived from the bark of the Pacific yew tree.

So before you get to the point of *needing* medicine in its concentrated form—in a pill, or a needle—why not get it from your dinner plate? When you eat Nature's medicine, you need less of the man-made kind.

I'm sure you can tell by now that I love whole plant foods. Once I found out about all the incredible things they can do, I never had to be talked into eating a big salad, or a bowl of brown rice. But if you need just a little more nudging to get excited, consider that:

THEY HAVE PRACTICALLY NO CALORIES: Whole plant foods are not only low-calorie, but your body knows how to use them efficiently, so they actually help to spur your metabolism. It's when you're eating refined foods that your system gets sludgy and heavy.

As I've been in the public eye since I was twelve, I try to stay in good shape. But there are healthy and unhealthy ways to do that (remember my diet pill problem?). So when I set my goal to lose some of the weight I didn't need in a way that wasn't going to hurt my body, I loved that I could fill up on whole grains and vegetables—and I mean really *fill up*—and stay on target! Plus, I had the most amazing energy. It was the exact opposite of my previous diets, which left me feeling weak and empty.

THEY ARE VERSATILE: As a cook, I love vegetables, whole grains, fruits, and seeds. They have a mind-blowing variety of colors, textures, flavors, and shapes. And when you multiply those qualities by all the different cooking styles, there are endless permutations of dinners waiting to be created! If you are already an artist in the kitchen, let's widen your palette. And if you're new to cooking altogether, whole plant foods will help you tap into your inner da Vinci.

THEY TASTE AMAZING: You may not believe this yet, especially if your brain has been hijacked by the processed food industry (which we'll talk about later), but all whole plant foods have complex, rich, and unique flavors. We've already determined that Nature isn't dumb . . . but she ain't boring, either.

After eating this way for just a few weeks, you will be able to perceive tastes you may not have registered, well, ever. A whole foods meal is much more sophisticated and satisfying than a Big Mac, or anything from a box.

I'm sure, by now, you get my point. Whole plants are good. They are here for us to eat. They are not weird "health" foods. They are *real* food.

In the next section, we move from complex carbohydrates to proteins—another vital nutrient I'm sure you've heard of—and we will investigate what it is, how much we need, and its various sources. Let's take a look.

High-Quality Protein

This includes:

- Organic, grass-fed, antibiotic-free foods derived from animals (meat, poultry, eggs, and fish, with the exception of dairy) and without added hormones.
- Organic beans and bean products.

This does *not* include:

- Processed meats, like conventional hot dogs, sausages, and cold cuts that include additives or added sugar.
- Meat or animal products from factory farms.

When I started the Body Ecology diet to regain my health, I was surprised and delighted that meat wasn't a total no-no. I like meat, and so does Cory; we didn't want to get rid of it completely. But I did make two big changes in my meat consumption: I had to *increase* the quality and *decrease* the quantity.

INCREASE THE QUALITY: This is really important. On page 60, we'll talk more in depth about factory-farmed meat and all of its problems, but this is the takeaway: If you're going to eat meat, it *must* be organic, grass-fed beef, pork, or lamb. This means it contains neither antibiotics nor added hormones, and that the animal ate its proper food. Chicken should be free-range and also free of antibiotics. Ditto eggs. Fish should be wild, and not farm-raised.

This is critical. The crappy stuff in factory-farmed meat leads to all kinds of nasty modern ailments. You can do a million good things for your health, and if you continue to eat factory-farmed meat, you will hurt yourself and any progress you've made. *It's that bad.*

Look, I know—buying high-quality meat is more expensive, and I don't want to dismiss that concern. But remember: You will be eating less of it, and enjoying it more. If you need to skimp elsewhere, like not buying 100 percent organic vegetables all the time, that's okay; you get fewer toxins from vegetables than you do from conventional meat. Hopefully your food bill will also balance out over time, after you've stocked your pantry with your awesome new ingredients and you're regularly cooking delicious grains, vegetables, and moderate amounts of meat.

This is about your health and your family's health, so it's a priority. If the organic meat is too expensive, make it a twice-weekly treat and start cooking more beans, which are very cheap, especially when you buy them dried and in bulk. Your wallet, your body, and your taste buds will thank you.

DECREASE THE QUANTITY: The United States is addicted to meat. And that causes lots of problems. Now, instead of making meat the central point of interest on my plate, it's just a small portion of my meal, sharing the spotlight with lots of vegetables, grains, and other plant-based foods. And I'm fine with that. The amount of meat on my plate makes up only 10 to 20 percent of my entire meal—that's it.

When I started cooking this way, I was surprised at how satisfying it was. But then I learned that it's how Asian and African cultures have eaten meat through the ages—as a special treat, not an everyday privilege. Heck, it's how Western cultures ate before we got so rich and meat-crazy. You just don't need a ton of meat for it to do its job. Its nutrients—protein, fat, and minerals—don't have to come in big doses to be effective, and too much is actually detrimental. We Americans like to have more, more, MORE . . . but that doesn't work for your perfect body. Too much of *anything* pushes it out of balance, and that's not good.

These days, I don't eat meat at every meal. Sometimes I eat beans, or bean products, and my breakfast often has no protein at all. It works for me, and I recommend you try it. Think 80 to 90 percent plants, and 10 to 20 percent (animal or bean) protein, okay? If you reduce your meat intake, you'll find that you enjoy it even more.

BEANS

Almost every culture in the world eats beans—whether it's tofu in Japan, frijoles in Mexico, hummus in Israel, or lentils in France. They're little powerhouses. High in protein but also rich in complex carbohydrates and fiber, beans are cheap, delicious, and easy to cook. There are many varieties of beans grown in the United States alone, so there's no excuse not to find a variety you love. Beans contain no cholesterol and get this: They put nitrogen back into the soil, prepping it for more plant growth. They're Nature's little helpers!

TO MY VEGGIE FRIENDS: If you want to take this journey without eating meat or any animal products at all, that's great. All the vegan recipes in this book are marked, and many of the others can be easily converted with a tweak or two. A vegetarian or vegan version of this diet still has tons of complex carbs, fiber, antioxidants, and phytochemicals, and you can get all the protein you need from beans and bean products. However, it's very important to eat sea vegetables and lots of leafy greens to make sure you get plenty of minerals. The only thing that's hard to find on a modern plant-based diet is a consistent source of vitamin B12, so my vegan friends take it in a supplement. And no, this doesn't mean that a plant-based diet is fundamentally deficient; B12 comes from bacteria that we used to get from the soil (and animals still do), but vegetables these days don't get to market with dirt on them, so they don't contain enough of it! It's another example of how what is good for the earth is good for our bodies.

What is protein?

Protein is one of three "macronutrients" that the human body needs. The others are carbohydrates and fat. We need all three, in relatively large amounts, to stay alive. "*Micronutrients*" are the itty-bitty nutrients—vitamins and minerals—and we need them too, but in much tinier amounts.

What does protein do?

Protein builds major parts of your body: your cells, your muscles, the enzymes that break down your food, your neurons, your . . . *you*. When it comes to building or maintaining the structure of your body, protein is key. Carbohydrates provide the gasoline, but protein (plus some minerals) build the car.

But let's rewind a bit here . . .

All proteins are made up of *amino acids*. There are twenty amino acids, and they combine with one another in a mind-boggling number of ways to make different proteins. For instance, it is estimated that there are at least 100,000 different proteins in the human body alone . . . all made from those twenty amino acids!

Of those twenty, eleven amino acids are made by the body, but nine are not; we call them the nine *essential* amino acids, and they need to come from food. Back in the day, we thought that all nine essential amino acids had to be consumed in one food—or at least at one meal—for the body to make enough protein. But guess what? It turns out our perfect bodies know how to mix and match amino acids throughout the day, all by themselves. You don't see gorillas sitting around with amino acid calculators, do you?

How much protein do I need?

You might assume that you need a lot of protein to maintain your body's structure, but that's not actually true. You've been building your body—little by little—every day since you were conceived, so now you just need to maintain it, doing some repairs here and there, growing some hair, nails, blood, etc. You don't need tons of protein to do that.

However, if you're pregnant, you are in the baby-building business, and you will need more protein. Ditto if you are an athlete, or have a very physically rigorous job. But rest assured, when your perfect body needs more protein, you will naturally crave more of it. You can trust your body. How cool is that?

I say this because we live in a culture that tends to *worry* about protein. Mothers of vegetarian children are always wringing their hands about Susie not getting "enough protein." Low-carb dieters and Paleos down protein shakes, on top of three-egg and bacon breakfasts, "for the protein." We've gone a little nuts about protein.

But protein isn't that hard to get; almost every food has it. Yes, even broccoli! Vegetarian animals like elephants don't seem to have any trouble growing to the size of a house, so they must be getting enough protein from the plants they eat. You see, amino acids are everywhere, and our bodies know exactly how to combine them. In fact, in our society, it's practically impossible to have a protein deficiency. Do you know anyone who's ever had one?

I didn't think so.

So it's time to stop worrying about protein—at least, not getting enough of it. The truth is, we should worry about getting *too much* protein. Many of the diseases that we see in the Western world can be traced to an excess of protein, and animal protein in particular.

You see, your body can't store excess protein, so it doesn't make sense to stock up on it. And when you've eaten too much, it converts back into amino acids. Too much acid of any kind causes your body to offer up minerals to balance it. These minerals come from your blood and then from your bones, so excess protein is a big factor in osteoporosis. Too much acid can also hurt the liver and kidneys. Excess animal protein has also been connected to different types of cancer.[3] Too much can promote gout, dehydration, and weight gain. In fact, the longest living peoples in the world eat lots of complex carbs and relatively little protein, choosing beans over meat most of the time.[4]

When it comes to protein, enough is enough. Let's consider it in light of the Three Concepts.

1. Are high-quality proteins whole?

Although they are parts of a bigger entity, we can consider cuts of meat whole, as long as they're not processed beyond that. Beans are whole.

2. Do high-quality proteins cause inflammation?

In general, no. Organic poultry, wild fish, and organic eggs do not cause inflammation. You see, cows, chickens, sheep, and pigs that eat what they are designed to (grass and other natural stuff) have a more balanced ratio of omega-6 to omega-3 fatty acids than conventional livestock. This is critical because as the ratio gets wider—with factory-farmed animals—inflammation follows. Turns out animals are what they eat too!

Even grass-fed red meat, however, can cause an inflammatory response. So if you eat red meat, make sure not to eat too much of it and to rotate it with other animal proteins or with beans, which don't cause inflammation. In fact, beans have natural anti-inflammatory properties. Remember: They're whole plant foods!

OMEGA WHAT? Along with carbohydrates and protein, fat is one of the three macro-nutrients and—like protein—breaks down into acids, which we call *fatty acids*. The human body makes almost all of these acids itself, but there are two that we can get only from food: omega-3 and omega-6, otherwise known as the essential fatty acids.

Omega-3s are critical to brain and heart health, and although they come from a variety of different sources, they are most abundantly found in the oils from very small fish like sardines and wild-caught Alaskan salmon.* These fatty acids are also found in flax, chia, and hemp seeds, and in much smaller amounts in leafy greens, cabbages, beans, and even winter squash.

Although omega-6 fatty acids also have some health benefits, eating too many of them makes those benefits disappear and problems—like heart disease—follow. You see, omega-6s are especially abundant in vegetable oils such as corn, safflower, and soy, and therefore, we end up getting them in many fried, fast, and processed foods. Omega-6s are also found in poultry, eggs, nuts, and avocados. An overabundance of omega-6s—compared to -3s—are in factory-farmed meats because the animals are eating imbalanced diets. And when there are too many omega-6s drowning out the omega-3s, a lot of inflammation occurs. The ratio of omega-3s to -6s should be relatively close—almost even—but in refined vegetable oils and badly nourished livestock, it's far from it.

3.   *Is high-quality protein good for gut bacteria?*

Meat gets broken down in our guts by certain bile-eating microbes, so meat eaters tend to develop more of those bacteria. In general, meat is not good for your microbiome *if all you eat is meat.* And let's face it: We all have an uncle who eats almost nothing but. But if you eat a moderate amount of organic animal protein in conjunction with lots of fiber-rich vegetables, grains, and fermented foods (see page 42), your gut bacteria should be varied and strong. The real gut problems begin when meat is full of antibiotics, which we will look at a little later.

*   Other fatty fish tend to contain too much mercury and other industrial toxins to make them wise choices as your source of omega-3s.

Beans are excellent for your bacteria. The bacteria love the fiber, and the special sugars in beans are such gut-favorites that they start throwing fart parties when they eat them! If you want to avoid that, soak dried beans before cooking and remember to chew them well; you'll start digesting them in your mouth and break down those special sugars *before* your critters can.

IS SOY SAFE?

Yes and no. Soybeans that are organic and whole (or have been only minimally processed) are not only safe, they are really, *really* good for you. Soy is a great source of protein, is high in antioxidants, and even has tumor-blocking properties. East Asian communities have consumed soy for thousands of years and have some of the longest life spans, with the fewest chronic diseases, in the world.

You may have also heard that soybeans contain phytoestrogens, plant-based compounds that mimic female hormones. Some people get freaked out about phytoestrogens because excess estrogen has been linked to breast cancer and other hormone-driven cancers in women. It has also been linked to enlarged breast tissue in men.

So let's address this: First, it's important to understand that phytoestrogens are much, much weaker than the hormones your body makes, or what you may be getting from drinking a glass of cow's milk (containing animal-created estrogen). So unless you're eating a ridiculous amount of soy, the estrogen issue shouldn't raise alarms.

That said, it's easier to eat a ridiculous amount of soy than you might think: Soy compounds—hiding behind names like isoflavones, soy protein isolates, or hydrolyzed soy—show up in a huge percentage of this country's run-of-the-mill processed foods. The farming of soybeans is subsidized in the United States, so we have a lot of cheap soy and we are putting it into just about everything. Add to that soy "milks," "cheeses," and "ice creams," and we've traveled far from Asia and the whole soybean and are gorging on a lot of processed soy. This is why it's easy to ingest too many phytoestrogens.

Back to the good news: In moderate amounts, soy's plant-based estrogens actually seem to help us by blocking some of our estrogen receptors, making sure we don't get too much of the human or animal version of the hormone. Instead of increasing our risk of breast cancer, soybeans apparently reduce it, especially in women who have never had the disease. Other foods containing phytoestrogens? Flax seeds, sesame seeds, garlic, alfalfa sprouts, multigrain bread, and dried apricots.

As always, we need to keep it simple: Get your soy from whole soybeans, like organic edamame, and minimally processed foods, like organic tofu and tempeh—both of which are so simple you can make them in your kitchen. Organic soy sauce, tamari (a wheat-free soy sauce), and miso are also fine.

It's okay to eat some processed soy products in order to ease your transition away from dairy, but please be moderate with them.

Sea Vegetables (a.k.a. Seaweed)

I . Love. Seaweed.

I know that sounds weird, but ever since I was introduced to eating the veggies that grow under-water, I have slowly fallen in love with them. And even better, seaweed loves me. These are some of the most powerful foods on the planet. They are PACKED with minerals and are good for us in many different ways.

For thousands of years, coastal cultures all over the world have eaten seaweed. No matter how novel or weird they seem to you and me, these are not new foods. Heck, we eat *animals* from the sea—so why not the plants?

There are roughly thirty types of edible sea vegetables, but the ones you'll find in the health-food store are:

- Arame (cooked with vegetables, or tossed in a salad)
- Hijiki, sometimes spelled "hiziki" (cooked with vegetables)
- Kombu/Kelp (used in bean dishes, or dried as a condiment)
- Wakame (used in soups, or eaten raw, with other vegetables)
- Nori (sold in sheets, and rolled into sushi rolls)
- Dulse (dried, as a condiment)
- Agar agar (used as a gelatin substitute)

If you eat at Japanese restaurants, you've already tasted wakame in miso soup and nori when it's wrapped around a sushi roll. If you're wary of jumping too deep into the world of sea vegetables, start with lunch at a Japanese restaurant and see what you think. Let's think about sea vegetables as they relate to the Three Concepts.

1. *Are sea vegetables whole?*

Yes.

2.   *Do sea vegetables cause inflammation?*

Absolutely not. Sea vegetables are naturally alkalizing, so they are powerful anti-inflammatories. They are also antiviral and prevent excess clotting of the blood. And did I mention that they lower cholesterol, and help block tumor growth?

ACID/ALKALINE BALANCE: Remember that week in high school chemistry class, when you learned how to determine whether something was more acidic or more alkaline by burning it and testing its ash? Well, different substances, whether consumed by fire or by your body, leave behind an acidic or an alkaline residue. This matters because our blood has a pH of roughly 7.4, so our natural, internal "balance" is slightly alkaline. If health is one long balancing act, alkalinity is the center of our body's inner teeter-totter.

Now, this doesn't mean we stay away from acid-forming foods altogether, but it does mean we should choose alkaline-forming foods 70 to 80 percent of the time. And of the acid-forming foods we eat, the milder ones are best. Here is a list of where some foods fall on the alkaline/acid spectrum:

Alkaline-forming foods: Lucky for us, there are many. Most vegetables, all sea vegetables, many fruits, and a handful of whole grains are naturally alkalizing, as are sea salt, miso, and good-quality soy sauce.

Mildly acid-forming foods: These include fish, eggs, some whole grains, some fruits, fruit juices, and non-dairy "milks."

Acid-forming foods that nudge the teeter-totter a little more: These include chocolate, coffee, and white flour.

Strongly acid-forming foods, and those that really tip the teeter-totter: These include meat, dairy, and highly processed foods, which is yet another reason to eliminate them. Eat very few of them or—in the case of meat—consume them with lots of veggies.

3.   *Are sea vegetables good for gut bacteria?*

Yes. In fact, seaweeds introduce unique and powerful bacteria to the mix of critters in your gut, and many seaweeds help soothe and support the lining of the intestine.[5]

WHAT ARE MINERALS?

Minerals are microscopic metals and other compounds found in nature. Remember the periodic table of elements? It includes gases, minerals, and metals like copper, magnesium, calcium, phosphorus, and iron. These are some of what we call "dietary minerals," which show up in food.

Minerals are also critical to your health. They facilitate almost every major process in the body, from muscle contraction to regulating blood pressure to forming and strengthening your bones. And what's more, minerals make for beautiful skin, lustrous hair, and diamond-hard nails! You'd be a downright wreck without your minerals.

We don't require a ton of minerals to reap all their sweet benefits—like I said, they're microscopic—but modern agriculture has depleted our soil over the years, reducing its mineral content. The good news is that we haven't yet managed to de-mineralize the sea, so seaweed comes complete with a lovely mix of available minerals. In fact, sea vegetables are quite possibly the most concentrated source of minerals that humans have access to. One ounce of hijiki has *fourteen times* more calcium than an ounce of milk—and it's a form of calcium that we can absorb easily.*

More good news about sea vegetables

SEAWEED HAS A SUPERPOWER: It gets rid of radioactivity. You heard me. Sea vegetables bind with radioactive isotopes in your body—from X-rays or other sources—and *discharges* them. It does the same thing with heavy metals, like lead and mercury. And believe me, you don't want to be messing with excess radiation or heavy metals; they are both cancer-causing and downright toxic. Thank goodness for sea vegetables!

---

* See the upcoming section on dairy to see how milk holds up in the calcium department. Spoiler alert: NOT SO GOOD.

Fermented Foods

Fermented foods have been consumed by almost every human culture we know of. The earliest records of fermentation reach back 8,000 years to the Middle East, so it's seriously old school. Most of us, however, born into a modern, industrialized, and fast-food world, have little or no experience of fermented foods on our family table. And when you look at the arc of human history, that's just weird.

Fermentation began as a way of preserving foods, before we had refrigerators. You see, when a food is salted or immersed in salty brine, it is protected from many food-borne pathogens. But it gets better: The salt favors a certain bacteria, lactobacillus, which feeds on the sugars of the food and creates lactic acid. Lactic acid is not only a natural preservative, it increases the vitamin content and digestibility of food, so fermented foods are super nutritious. Lactobacillus is also one of the really good critters in your gut, so eating fermented foods helps support your healthy microbiome.

When I say fermented foods, I mean: cultured vegetables and unpasteurized pickles, a.k.a. pickled vegetables, made with salt,* as well as unpasteurized miso and unpasteurized soy sauce. (Although tempeh, cheese, and yogurt are also fermented, you cannot find unpasteurized versions of them in American stores—it's the law.)

And pasteurization matters. In 1864, scientist Louis Pasteur discovered that heating wine and beer killed off the bacteria that would turn them sour. This process was introduced to many foods, fermented and otherwise. And that's not a bad thing; in a country with a huge food industry, where perishable items are being shipped long distances in less-than-sterile environments, pasteurization has made our overall food supply much safer. The problem is that pasteurizing also kills *good* bacteria—exactly the critters we want to keep!

So, when it comes to cultured vegetables, pickles, and miso, we must make sure to buy unpasteurized versions, from health-food stores or online. Or, you can make our own! They're easy and delicious. (See some introductory recipes, starting on page 211.)

So let's check in with our three questions:

1.   *Are fermented foods whole?*

Yes. They are made from whole foods.

2.   *Do fermented foods cause inflammation?*

No. They are decidedly anti-inflammatory. And some even contain superpowers: For instance, miso has been found to fend off radiation, suppress tumor growth, and, even though it's made with salt

---

* Some pickles are made with vinegar and although they are tasty, they do not have the same health benefits.

(sea salt, which contains a ton more minerals than table salt), it can help keep blood pressure down.[6]

3.   Are fermented foods good for gut bacteria?

With fermented foods, your minuscule friends win the lottery. Eating cultured vegetables, pickles, and miso soup on a regular basis is the nicest thing you can do for your gut. And as you know by now, that means it's good for your immunity and your health in every other way. Pickle, anyone?

FERMENTED FOODS: *The World Tour*

Korea: Kimchi. **Germany:** Sauerkraut. **Scandinavia:** Pickled Herring. **Japan:** Miso, Natto. **Indonesia:** Tempeh. **France:** Unpasteurized Cheese. **Greece:** Yogurt. **Peru:** Chicha. **Mexico:** Pulque. **China:** Kombucha. **Russia:** Kefir, Kvass.

Tia Tip: I often make the recipe for cultured vegetables in this book (page 211), which comes from *The Body Ecology Diet*. I love it. If I'm feeling under the weather, or if Cree comes home with a bug, I make sure to eat at least a tablespoon of cultured vegetables at every meal—it's the best illness prevention you'll find in your fridge. But one thing you should know: Cultured vegetables can stink, in a garlicky, pickle-y way. Not all fermented foods smell so strong, but homemade ones often do.

But that doesn't stop me. Recently, I took a big Tupperware to the set of the show *Instant Mom* and was happily snacking away when a producer from the network came in to watch us work. Now, that's normally all well and good, *except* that this time she wanted to speak to me. I thought, *"Crap!* I just ate cultured cabbage!" I knew I still had the whiff of it on me. As I shook her hand, I frantically explained before she could assume I'd farted! HA!

Honestly, not all cultured vegetables can clear a room. Buy some unpasteurized sauerkraut or unpasteurized organic dill pickles to get you into the swing of things; they don't have a strong smell. After a while you'll get into the more creative (and aromatic) possibilities. And remember: Once your homemade cultured vegetables have fermented, they can be kept in the fridge with a closed lid and no one will be the wiser. Personally, I've come to have a lot of affection for that smell, but it can be an adjustment.

These days, fermented foods are getting a lot of attention because they are ridiculously healthy; they're not considered that weird anymore, and they are truly tasty to boot. So give them a whirl—you might find you love how they taste and how, more importantly, they make you feel.

Safer Sweets

Life is supposed to be sweet. As someone with a pronounced sweet tooth, I couldn't go on without a treat here and there. Good-quality sweets are relaxing and necessary for the soul—not to mention one's sense of humor. Just because you're eating healthier food doesn't mean you have to give them up.

The issue with most of the sugar we eat is how refined it is. In the next section, we are going to be talking about white sugar and other highly refined carbohydrates; as with all foods, the less refined, the better. Lucky for us, there are a ton of foods that are fantastically sweet in their whole form. Fruits, squashes, cooked onions, sweet potatoes, and even carrots will taste extra luscious to you *after* you get off white sugar. If you haven't given refined sugar the heave-ho yet, your taste buds are still acclimated to an unnatural level of sweetness and your brain sends out pleasure chemicals only when you eat the strong stuff. This might make fruits and veggies seem a little boring *now,* but it won't take long for your body to recalibrate and for you to experience the gorgeous, deep, and subtle pleasures of . . . a yam!

When we want to give our whole foods an extra kick, we can use sweeteners that have been minimally processed—and in moderate amounts. That's key. Yes, life should and will be sweet, but you shouldn't be bathing in a tub of brown rice syrup—it's not a healthy alternative if you overdo it. Of course, when you're quitting white sugar, you can use more alternative sweeteners to deal with your cravings (see pages 45–46 for nourishing options that'll still satisfy your withdrawal urges), but we're not here to replace one bad habit with another. A dessert here and there made with rice syrup and non-dairy chocolate is fine. Forgoing whole foods for nightly pancake dinners—even if you're using organic maple syrup—is not.

Here's the thing: Most of the sweeteners we use are processed in some way—whether through fermentation, reduction, or other means—to achieve their intense taste. If you've ever tasted the subtle sweetness of maple sap straight from the tree, you know how weak it is compared to maple syrup. Our job is to choose the sweeteners that land most softly on the human body. And if you are wrestling with Candida or have any other condition that is exacerbated by sugar, stick to yams and carrots until you've got it under control.

So let's ask our three questions:

1. *Are safer sweets whole?*

Yes and no. Squash, onions, and other sweet vegetables are whole. Fruits are whole. Any syrup or processed sweet is not.

2. Do safer sweets cause inflammation?

Again, the sweet whole plant foods (onions, squash, etc.) do not cause inflammation. In fact, most are anti-inflammatory. Many fruits contain anti-inflammatory compounds, too. Stevia—the one sugar replacement on our list that is actually *not* a sugar—does not cause inflammation.

The rest of the sweeteners below are generally safe, but if you gorge on any of them, eating large amounts on a regular basis, inflammation may follow. So go easy. Even though maple syrup, honey, and brown rice syrup have some nutritional benefits—even anti-inflammatory ones—they are, ultimately, sugar. And too much sugar causes inflammation.

3. Are safer sweets good for gut bacteria?

As with most things, if it's coming from a whole food, fear not! Sweet vegetables, whole fruits, and other whole foods are just fine. With respect to sweeteners, it's all about refinement: The more highly refined a sugar, the more unstable it makes your gut bacteria and the more the bad critters binge on it. That's why people with gut issues should stay away from sugar—even the less refined options. However, if you're in good health and eating a diet with lots of vegetables, grains, and other whole plants, a little natural sweetener will go down just fine.

Stevia has been found to depress the growth of certain good bacteria, but not others,[7] so it's a bit of a mixed bag.

SAFER SWEETS FOR REGULAR USE:

STEVIA: I was introduced to stevia by *The Body Ecology Diet*. For those people looking to starve Candida and other yeasts in the body, it is crucial that they eat no refined sugars at all. That means no brown rice syrup, no maple, no coconut sugar. No nuthin'.

But, even though it tastes extremely sweet, stevia isn't actually a sugar. Derived from an herb, stevia has no calories and no carbohydrates, so it is perfect for people with Candida or diabetes. You can use stevia in tea, coffee, or a grown-up party drink. It is not great for baking, however, and I wouldn't want to pour stevia all over a stack of pancakes. But that's just me. Try it for yourself!

BROWN RICE SYRUP: This is made from brown rice that's been slowly fermented. The gooey, sweet syrup that results consists of approximately 60 percent complex carbohydrates. Remember, those are the *slow* carbs! So even though brown rice syrup is very sweet, it is absorbed into your blood slowly compared to white sugar. It's one of my favorite sweetener alternatives.

MAPLE SYRUP: This sweet, amber fluid has more simple carbohydrates (fast carbs) than brown rice syrup, but it also contains minerals that give the syrup its brown color. These minerals help you metabolize the maple syrup's sugar, so you don't become depleted.

DATE SUGAR: This sweetener consists of ground-up dehydrated dates, so it's the pulverized version of a whole food. Which sounds great, but as soon as a whole food is pulverized, it is absorbed much more quickly into the bloodstream. This means that you might still get that sugar high and crash. Date sugar can be a tasty substitution in some recipes but it has a particular taste, so try it before combining it with other ingredients. You can also purchase date syrup; it has a similar taste, but can be poured.

HONEY: Lovely honey comes straight to us from the bees. Honey is antimicrobial, and raw honey contains antioxidants, minerals, trace enzymes, and other beneficial things. Used as a sweetener for much of human history, honey—consumed in moderation—is one of Nature's miracle foods. That said, I sometimes find it too sweet and don't use it that much in my cooking.

TO USE HERE AND THERE:

AGAVE SYRUP: This comes from the agave cactus and is pretty highly refined, but many people can ingest it without experiencing the addictive roller coaster of white sugar. But go easy. I would choose brown rice syrup over agave.

COCONUT SUGAR: This is like the maple sugar of the tropics. Coconut palm trees are tapped for their sap, which is reduced into a syrup and then dried. It still contains some antioxidants, fiber, and even amino acids. That said, when I'm trying to kick white sugar (it creeps into my diet every once in a while), I give up coconut and palm sugars too. Although I use coconut sugar in a handful of the sweeter recipes in this book, coconut and palm sugar feel the most like treats of all the sweeteners on this list, and too much of them can leave me craving more.

PALM SUGAR: These crystals also come from the dehydrated sap of the palm tree, but not the coconut palm. Palm sugar has similar qualities, both good and bad, to coconut sugar.

MOLASSES: You won't find any recipes in this book using molasses, but it's a sweetener that's been around for a long time and is used primarily in baking. Made from the syrup left over from the sugar refining process, molasses contains, among other minerals, iron, calcium, and magnesium, which help to balance its simple carbohydrates. It also has a very concentrated, intense flavor, so try it and see what you think.

So that's it: Foods that heal. Foods that are friendly to our bodies. I encourage you to explore them and see what you like! If these foods seem strange to you, remember that your body *knows* them; your ancestors ate them and, in fact, your DNA was built on them. You MUST try them for your health, but once you get into the groove, it won't be a chore. Eating these foods is natural, even innate. By eating them, you're *coming home*.

THE POWER OF FOOD

Now, let's take a look at the foods that we want to start steering away from, gently. Think of them simply as foods that are rough on your health; they make your perfect body work too hard in order to maintain balance. Some of them may come as a surprise, while others you know, in your gut, aren't working for you.

They are:

- Sugar and Other Highly Refined Carbohydrates
- Dairy Foods
- Factory-Farmed Meats
- Processed and Fast Foods
- Refined Oils and Refined Salts

Again, we look at each category through the lens of our Three Concepts:

1. *Is it whole?*
2. *Does it cause inflammation?*
3. *Is it good for your gut bacteria?*

Sugar and Other Highly Refined Carbohydrates

When I talk about sugar, I mean highly refined sugar: the crystals—white or brown—that are made from sugarcane or beets. They have a few aliases: brown sugar, raw sugar, evaporated cane juice, turbinado sugar, Florida Crystals, and just about anything ending with "ose," as in sucrose, dextrose, or maltose. "Sugar" also refers to high-fructose corn syrup, which sounds all nice and homey, like you're eating corn from a farm, but may be the worst of them all.

HIGH-FRUCTOSE HELL: If white sugar weren't bad enough, a new sweetener, high-fructose corn syrup (HFCS), hit the scene in the early 1970s. Over the last forty-plus years, it has crept into a huge percentage of sodas, cereals, breads, and even salad dressings. Here in the United States, we eat more HFCS than any other country in the world—upward of fifty-five pounds, per person, per year. And that's *in addition to* all other refined sugars.

What's the problem? Well, studies have shown that HFCS breaks down in the body quite differently than sucrose. When rats were given food laced with HFCS, they got fatter and gained weight more quickly than rats given food that contained sucrose (white sugar). Even worse, the weight they gained showed up around their little middles—that's the dangerous, you-might-have-a-heart-attack fat connected to metabolic syndrome.[8] HFCS has also been shown to raise triglycerides,[9] also a big factor in heart disease. Yikes.

But here's the kicker: HFCS causes your body to secrete fewer hormones that send the message that you're full and that make you feel satisfied—so you just keep eating.[10] Our ballooning obesity rates may be driven in part by the "special" qualities of high-fructose corn syrup. *All* refined sugar is hard on the body, but HFCS may be in a category all by itself.

And by highly refined carbohydrates, I mean white flour and all the things it's made into: bread, pasta, cupcakes, bagels, cookies, crackers . . . you name it. The yummy stuff! I also mean any grain that's been stripped of everything except its carbohydrate, like white rice. White-flour products and white rice basically behave just like sugar in your body, which is why we're looking at sugar and refined carbohydrates together.

Let's see how they shake down:

1.   *Are sugar and refined carbs whole?*

Far from it.

Think of it this way: Your body can handle eating a whole beet or gnawing on a piece of sugarcane. Both of these foods, left intact, deliver fiber, minerals, and vitamins *along* with their sugar. And that's great, because to metabolize the sugar properly, your body needs all of those other components. So understand: There's nothing wrong with natural sugars, which can be found in all complex carbohydrates. When they come *inside* whole foods, sugars are the best fuel there is for the human body.

Go sugar!

But when the beet or the sugarcane is stripped of all its other good stuff and is left just a bunch of bleached crystals, it becomes a *simple* carbohydrate, and your body isn't designed to handle it very well. It makes a valiant effort—raising your blood sugar, secreting lots of insulin, giving up minerals from your bloodstream—to balance this hit, but no matter how hard your body works, it ends up losing the sugar game.

It's the same deal with white flour, which is the pure carbohydrate taken from a whole wheat berry, stripped of its fiber, germ, minerals, and vitamins. Ditto white rice and white rice flour. These pure carbohydrates put your body on a similar roller coaster.*

Yes, your body works perfectly, but when you eat highly refined foods, you are constantly putting yourself under stress, and this quickly takes its toll. Like a drug addict, you come away depleted and weakened by powerful white crystals, or white powder. If we were honest with ourselves, we would categorize sugar and white flour as drugs, not foods.

> **SWEET CREE:** I find that when I introduce sugar into my body after staying away from it for a while, it's amazing how exhausted and sluggish I become! But I really see its impact on my son's personality. Whenever Cree's on sugar, he starts to act like a different person, like he's possessed. He has tons of energy, bounces off the walls, gets aggressive, and then crashes, hard. It's crazy. Cory and I have learned to put two and two together. If he's being extra nutty, the first thing we think is: "He stayed over at Grandma's this weekend . . . What did he eat?" And then my mother will confess that she gave him cookies and ice cream. That was a huge wake-up call for me: realizing not only how sugar affects *my* body, but how it affects my son's.

2.   *Do sugar and highly refined carbs cause inflammation?*

You betcha. They are real baddies, in this department.

The inflammation caused by refined carbs is so apparent that scientists have recently been pointing at sugar and white flour as the chief underlying dietary factors in obesity, diabetes, insulin resistance, high blood pressure, kidney disease, and even heart disease. These conditions often show up in the same person as one big dangerous package called "metabolic syndrome." And what connects the dots between these health conditions? Inflammation. We used to think that meat played the biggest role in heart disease, but the newest research shows that the chief culprit behind a heart attack may be not meat . . . but *sugar*.[11]

---

* Whole-grain flours keep all their bits and pieces so are much healthier than white flour, but they still aren't whole foods. See the sidebar "What about Flour?" on page 28.

A SHORT, SWEET HISTORY: In the West, we have had access to white sugar for only 500 years, and for the first 400, we cherished it as a rare luxury. It's only in the last century that we've gone from eating four pounds of sugar per year to over a hundred![12] And remember: Homo sapiens have been around for over 200,000 years, so that's a huge increase over a very short period of time. Before the sixteenth century, you might have enjoyed a sweet lick of honey here and there or baked it into a holiday treat, but sugar in its crystallized form, inside and on top of so many foods around us, is an entirely new phenomenon. No wonder it's doing so much damage—we're just not designed for it.

3.   *Are sugar and highly refined carbs good for your gut bacteria?*

No. They weaken your friendly critters. Not only that, the bad guys *love* sugar and other refined carbs. That's why I got into so much trouble; my gut bacteria were already out of whack because of all the antibiotics I had taken, and by eating sugary processed foods, I was offering a Thanksgiving feast to my bad bacteria three times a day. My Candida loved it! What's the first thing a Candida sufferer is told to give up? You guessed it: sugar.

More Bad News about Sugar and Highly Refined Carbs

THEY MAKE YOU CRAZY: Because they are converted to blood sugar so quickly, sugar and white flour cause your body to secrete too much insulin. To fix that, your poor body secretes another hormone called anti-insulin. Because your glands work in harmony, this roller coaster of hormone production messes with *all* your hormones—and your moods.

Sugar and bread addicts may recognize this cycle: Some days, you go up and down, cycling between crying and yelling. Your PMS is cranked up to eleven. Perhaps you experience depression. You may not recognize yet that your emotional life is being controlled by the sweet and baked stuff, but when you go off it for as few as ten days, you'll see what I mean. Life is much more balanced and peaceful after you kick that junk out the door.

HIGHLY REFINED CARBS ARE ADDICTIVE: If you've tried to give up sugar and/or white flour before, you've probably found it really hard. I've been there. I've said it before, but it bears repeating: Sugar is so highly refined that it acts more like a drug in your brain than a normal food. Ditto white flour, for many people.

Here's how it works: Highly refined carbohydrates work on a part of your brain that secretes plea-sure chemicals, so when you eat them, you get more than an instant hit of energy. You get a dose of your own, homemade happy pills . . . followed by a crash. So kicking sugar and white flour can also mean going through withdrawal. That's your first sign that something in your diet isn't normal. You weren't designed to get *high* when you eat, and whole foods don't elicit that response. Ask yourself: When was the last time you had a desperate *craving* for a carrot? Or cried over not having a bowl of barley? There's a very real, natural pleasure in eating, but if cavewomen were all running around like drugged-out, greedy, cranky junkies, the human race probably wouldn't have made it this far.

Tia Tip: Find a friend who wants to get off the white stuff with you, so you can hold each other's hands during the rough spots. I'm sure you'll find a pal like this easily!

HIGHLY REFINED CARBS CAN MAKE YOU GAIN WEIGHT: Remember that sugar and white flour are stripped of all their fiber, minerals, and vitamins. They are pure, high-calorie energy—like a shot in the arm. That's why runners eat simple carbs in the middle of a race, when their bodies are burning crazy amounts of energy.

But for the rest of us, this quick hit is not so great. We're not running marathons at the office—or even on the set of a TV show—and our bodies are stationary much of the time. With this kind of lifestyle, fast, simple carbs like sugar and white flour pump our blood sugar too high. This causes our bodies to create lots of insulin in order to mop up all that sugar. And do you know what the biggest mechanism behind fat storage is? Not the amount of calories you eat, but how much *insulin* those calories cause you to secrete. The more insulin you produce, the more fat you store. So simple carbs mean high insulin, which means weight gain.

On the other hand, when you eat a complex or slow carb (a whole food), your blood sugar rises slowly, which causes much less insulin to be secreted by your pancreas. And that means your body actually uses the food efficiently—over time—instead of storing it as excess. Not only do complex carbs give you a smoother, happier, healthier ride, they keep your blood sugar and insulin in balance. Less insulin means less fat.

Dairy Foods

Ah, dairy. Nature's perfect food. We're about to take a careful look at that widely held belief, and you may be surprised by what we learn about milk, cheese, yogurt, and other dairy products from a cow, goat, or sheep.

1. *Is dairy a whole food?*

Yes, dairy is a whole food. But it's time to ask yourself: Is it a whole food that is right for *you?* Nature is a precise force: When you plant a rose seed, only a rose will grow out of it—there isn't a crapshoot determining what kind of flower the seed will produce. Similarly, every female mammal produces a perfect and specific milk for her offspring. Baby whales need whale's milk. Piglets need pig's milk. And humans need human milk. Each is tailor-made for the species that produces it: For instance, the average female calf grows to over 400 pounds in her first *eight months*. Cow's milk is high in protein, minerals, and growth hormones—perfect for the bones, muscles, and turbo-charged physical growth of a calf. Meanwhile, human babies grow to only twenty or twenty-five pounds in their first year, and the biggest part of the baby's body is the head. Human milk is much higher in carbohydrates and fat than cow's milk in order to stimulate and grow the human brain.

Every type of milk contains the basic nutrients of protein, fat, carbohydrates, vitamins, and minerals, but Nature fits these pieces together differently for each species. It's precise. And that matters.

2. *Does dairy cause inflammation?*

Yes. Dairy causes lots of inflammation.

But it took me a while to really understand this. I had heard a lot of people talking about how we shouldn't be eating dairy, but when a Harvard-educated physician—my doctor—told me I needed to stay away from it, I finally listened.

And she was warning me about inflammation. Turns out that a protein in dairy—casein—is one of the most inflammatory foods there is for the human body. Our bodies just don't recognize the casein in cow's milk, so red flags go up when it's introduced. The casein in human milk is structured a little differently, so our bodies can digest it. With cow's milk, not so much.

So if you're eating dairy at breakfast, lunch, and dinner, you are likely experiencing chronic inflammation, and some savvy doctors are beginning to connect these dots. It's not unheard of for medical professionals who specialize in arthritis, skin disorders, allergies, and even autoimmune diseases to tell their patients to cool it with the dairy, just like mine did. A chronic runny nose, for instance, can often be dried up by kicking dairy.

But it doesn't take bingeing on dairy to cause a nasty reaction; the alarm bells go off with just one serving. Try avoiding all dairy for a month and then drink a big ole glass of milk; your stuffy nose will convince you better than I can. As I've said, Nature is very precise, and your perfect body can detect cow's casein on even a microscopic level.

3.   *Is dairy good for gut bacteria?*

This is an interesting question. If you are lactose intolerant (which we'll get into), drinking a glass of milk will be painful because your gut no longer produces the enzyme to digest it. On the other hand, when dairy is fermented as in yogurt, cheese, or kefir, it tends to be digested more easily and even contains some friendly bacteria that may be good for you.

However, many dairy cows in this country are given antibiotics to treat mastitis—an infection in their udders from being overmilked. There are traces of antibiotics in American milk despite the milk being tested before it reaches us.[13] And as you know, that's bad news for your friendly microbiome.

So is dairy good for gut bacteria? Not especially. All the critters that come in homemade fermented dairy products are available in other fermented foods (like miso, cultured vegetables, and naturally fermented pickles), so when you weigh all the pros and cons, it's just not worth it.

More Bad News about Dairy

LACTOSE INTOLERANCE: We've looked at the protein called casein and how the body reacts to it, but casein is only the beginning. Cow's milk also contains lactose, a sugar, which is difficult for many, many people to digest.

This should be no surprise to any of my African American, Asian, and Latina readers who get bloated and gassy after a glass of milk. I certainly do! That's inflammation, too. Estimates differ slightly but among adults, roughly 50 percent of Latinos and 70 percent of African Americans experience lactose malabsorption. The rate is considered to be even higher in Asian adults.[14] That brings us to approximately 65 percent[15] of the world's population being lactose "intolerant"!

That term, therefore, is misleading: "Lactose intolerance" makes it sound like it's an abnormality, or even a problem of some kind. But when *two thirds* of the human race has the same issue, it's completely normal. And guess who else doesn't produce lactase after infancy?

Every single other mammal on the planet.

You see, no other mammals drink milk after they're weaned, let alone milk from another species. It's. Just. Not. Done. We are the only species that drinks milk after the toddler years. Kinda weird when you think about it.

So why do we do it?

Well, it seems that Western and Northern Europeans, at some point in their history, started producing lactase as adults through a genetic adaptation so that they could lean on their herds to survive. Animal milk was critical under harsh conditions and during times of famine. A few South Asian cultures have the same genetic variation.

But the rest of the world's major civilizations were built without dairy being central to their diets. China started drinking cow's milk only relatively recently (largely because of Western influence) as did Japan and Korea, and all those civilizations have strong, proud, and fascinating culinary histories—without dairy. The history of African food is epic, rich, and vibrant, too, and dairy cows are not a big part of that picture. So maybe the adaptation that allowed a few populations to digest lactose was a genetic bandage as opposed to an evolutionary leap. Perhaps "lactose intolerance" should be renamed "perfect bodies, working perfectly." And even if you have the ability to digest lactose, that doesn't mean that cow's (or goat's or sheep's) dairy is *good* for you. It still causes inflammation, and a host of other problems I will talk about in a minute.

So if you're lactose "intolerant," and you think that you're odd, or weak, or have a problem that needs fixing, think again.

I believe you're *lucky*.

DAIRY MAY NOT PREVENT OSTEOPOROSIS: Wait. *What?* Word on the street is that the calcium in milk protects us from osteoporosis.

This is where it gets funky, my friend, so take a deep breath. We have all been told—again and again—that in order to have strong bones, we must drink lots of milk. And because we've been getting this message our whole lives, it must be true, right? And if it's true, then countries where people drink little or no milk must have severe problems with osteoporosis . . . The women of Beijing must be breaking their hips just crossing the street, no?

Oh wait. They don't *get* osteoporosis at the rates we do.

You heard me: It turns out that the countries with the highest dairy consumption have the *highest* rates of osteoporosis. And the countries with the lowest dairy consumption? You guessed it. The best bones.[16] In a twelve-year Harvard study, using data from 78,000 women, those who drank three glasses of milk a day experienced more bone fractures than those who rarely drank milk.[17]

Which leads us to the fact that:

DAIRY MAY NOT DELIVER ALL ITS CALCIUM: Yes, technically dairy contains calcium. Lots of it. But it also contains lots of phosphorus, which interferes with your ability to absorb that calcium. You see, cow's milk was designed for a cow's gut, which works perfectly with that ratio of phosphorus to calcium. Yours may not. The members of the National Dairy Council aren't lying when they say that milk contains calcium, but they're not telling the whole truth, either. Milk may contain calcium but that doesn't mean you're *getting* it. Got it?

Remember, the National Dairy Council's only job is to sell dairy. That's it. They're not doctors. Or nutritionists. Or even scientists. They are a lobbying group, and state on the research area of their website that they're in the business of "fostering new research on . . . The quality, performance and safety of dairy foods and ingredients that will lead to *increased consumption of dairy*"[18] (italics mine). So that makes it pretty clear: They fund research that aims to find the benefits from dairy products—in order to sell more dairy.

I'm not trying to hit you over the head with this. I'm just saying that if you feel pressure to drink a daily glass of milk even if you don't love how it makes you feel—as if it's Nature's "perfect food"—you're not crazy. The pressure exists. And there's big money behind it: The dairy industry in this country is huge, generating tens of billions of dollars per year.

But back to your bones . . .

Dairy may even contribute to bone loss: Remember when we talked about protein in the last chapter, and how you can absorb too much of it? Well, dairy contains lots of protein, and after your body takes what it needs, the excess breaks down into its original amino acids. Too much acid is not balanced, so your body offers up minerals to neutralize it (neat trick!). And where do you get these minerals? First you pull them from your blood. Then you go to your mineral bank account . . . your bones.

Uh-oh.

Yep, it's true: Dairy consumption, over time, *may be one of the contributors to osteoporosis.*[19*] That's also why countries with the highest dairy consumption per capita have the highest osteoporosis rates.

> **SO WHERE DO I GET MY CALCIUM?** There are lots of foods that are rich in calcium, like sea vegetables, collard greens, broccoli, kale, soybeans (and tofu), bok choy, figs, oranges, sardines, canned salmon, white beans, okra, almonds, and sesame seeds. But honestly, the issue isn't so much getting calcium as it is *keeping* it. By abstaining from calcium thieves like dairy, excess meat, white sugar, and processed foods, your body will hang on to the calcium it gets from other sources.

DAIRY CONTAINS EXCESS HORMONES: Because it comes from an animal, dairy contains hormones. Strong hormones. Your average glass of milk contains estrogen and progesterone, to name a couple, and that's *before* the dairy industry adds more—like bovine growth hormone—to the mix!

Think about it: Dairy comes from nursing cows, most of which are pregnant (the average American dairy cow is pregnant *300 days per year*). And the later in the pregnancy, the more hormones the cow produces when milked.

---

* Too much protein of any kind breaks down into acids and can cause mineral loss. This is why moderation in meat consumption is important.

The thing about hormones is that you really don't need more than your body makes, in general. Extra plant-based estrogens can be helpful when menopause approaches, but otherwise trust that your perfect body knows how to juggle all your hormones gracefully. When extra hormones are introduced, especially animal hormones, your body struggles to process them. In one study, the milk of pregnant cows was shown to alter significantly the hormonal balance in all research subjects—men, women, and children alike.[20]

After a while, excess hormones can fuel big problems, like endometriosis (hello!). Excess sex hormones in particular contribute to breast, uterine, ovarian, and cervical cancers in women and prostate and testicular cancers in men. As if that wasn't bad enough, dairy—a food that is meant to turbocharge growth—contains something called "insulin-like growth factor 1," or IGF-1. IGF-1 is present in both cows and humans, and when we eat or drink dairy, our levels of IGF-1 rise. After rapid childhood development, this is a big problem, because IGF-1 not only fuels your body's growth, it feeds the growth and cell division of tumors. Studies conducted at Harvard Medical School showed that high IGF-1 levels in adults increase the risk of breast, prostate, and colorectal cancers.[21]

DAIRY IS ADDICTIVE: Like sugar, dairy can be hard to kick, and there's a good reason for that. The protein I mentioned earlier—casein—contains a protein fragment called "casomorphin." Casomorphin acts on your brain like junior-league morphine, attaching to your opiate receptors and making you feel *goooood*.

If you've ever seen a baby looking stoned at the boob, this makes sense; human casomorphins help babies relax and bond with Mommy and keep them coming back for more. But eventually, we grow teeth, start to eat solid foods, and get pleasure from all sorts of other things, like relationships, and playing with puppies . . .

And *CHEESE*! Haha.

Cheese, as dairy foods go, has the most concentrated amount of casein. Cheese is like milk, on *crack*. I hear it all the time: "I could give up milk, but never cheese!" And there's something to that; cheese is mildly addictive.

But fear not. I used to feel the same way. But kicking dairy won't have you freaking out like a junkie. You may miss it for a bit, but after a few weeks, it may start to seem like an odd thing to put in your body. Or even a little gross. You will feel pleasantly *detached*. Unless you're a baby, casomorphin is not actually supposed to be in your stomach.

Remember: Your body *knows*.

WOULD YOU LIKE SOME COFFEE WITH THAT CREAM AND SUGAR?

I'll take a pass. When I first started working on *The Game,* I was still in my unhealthy rut. I always needed a pick-me-up around two in the afternoon, so I would get myself a cup of coffee. No biggie. Everyone drinks coffee!

But we often had run-throughs around that time of day, rehearsing the whole show in front of producers and network executives. And I would get *so nervous*! And sure, it's normal to be nervous under those circumstances, but I'm talking panic attacks. And I kept thinking: "What is *wrong* with me? I know my lines, I'm prepared, why am I freaking out?" All it took was a little experimenting, and I found my answer: When I let go of my late afternoon latte, the nerves disappeared.

Are there situations in your life that feel out of control? Times when anxiety or fear take over? Caffeine may be stirring up those feelings, and you don't even know it.

Most people start using caffeine—often in soft drinks—as kids, and move on to coffee or strong tea as adults. Coffee tends to get a free pass in our culture, and it does have some beneficial properties, but it's far from a miracle drug; moderate to heavy coffee consumption has been shown to increase inflammation, specifically the inflammation that leads to heart disease.[22]

Now, I'm a big believer in green tea. It's chock-full of antioxidants and it gives me just enough caffeine to stay alert through any slump, without making me so jacked up that I get anxious, like I do on coffee.

Eighty-three percent of Americans drink coffee,[23] so if that includes you, if you haven't gone without it for a while, maybe now's the time to find out how you feel on green tea, or no caffeine at all. If you're a heavy coffee drinker, start slow—each week, replace one cup a day with tea until you're off the stuff completely. You've got nothing to lose but the jitters!

Processed and Fast Foods

You know the drill: If it's comes from a factory or a laboratory, it's processed. Chances are, when you reach into a bag or a box, you're eating a processed food.* Fast food means any restaurant that has a drive-through, or is part of a big chain. Yes, pizza counts. Let's take a look at these foods using the Three Concepts.

1.   Are processed and fast foods whole?

No. They are the definition of "not whole."

Although certain items at a fast food restaurant may be whole, like the veggies in a salad, the major menu favorites—burgers, buns, etc.—are generally made with processed ingredients.

That said, it's important to understand that most foods we eat are processed, a bit. To cook a food is to process it. However, there's a big difference between blending vegetables into a lovely autumn soup, and the acrobatics that go into making a Twinkie. Use your noggin—you know which one's which.

2.   Do processed foods cause inflammation?

Yes. When I ate my beloved Cheetos, I was absorbing dyes, stabilizers, artificial flavors and colors, and other chemicals used to make them. *Plus* highly refined salt and oil. Not to mention the absurd amount of herbicides and pesticides sprayed on the genetically modified corn that they're made from. With every Cheeto, I was introducing new, complicated, and toxic substances into my body that caused an inflammatory response.

So the bad news about processed foods is not just their "empty" calories, or the fact that they taste like salty cardboard; processed foods *cause chronic inflammation*. And you know by now that chronic inflammation leads to a host of other nasties, like obesity, diabetes, heart disease, autoimmune diseases, and metabolic syndrome, to name just a few.

To add insult to injury, our bodies become acclimated to these "foods." Going without nutrients starts to feel normal, as we quietly lose our vibrancy. So don't be deceived: Just because you don't feel sick after eating something doesn't mean it isn't doing damage.

3.   Are processed and fast foods good for gut bacteria?

Nope. They're downright dangerous.

Our gut bacteria have evolved alongside (and inside) humans, so they recognize the actual foods that we've eaten for millennia. Processed foods, as created by the modern food industry, have existed

---

* Although not always: Edamame and frozen—or dried—fruit come in bags!

only for the last seventy years, since the end of World War II. Not only are processed foods "foreign" to your gut critters, they are so full of unnatural substances that they tend to upset the overall balance in your intestines.

Tim Spector, a professor of genetic epidemiology at King's College London, decided to find out just how much gut bacteria was affected by fast food. Spector's twenty-three-year-old son, Tom, agreed to eat nothing but food from McDonald's for ten days. Spector and his fellow researchers tested Tom's gut bacteria before, after, and during the experiment. Prior to eating the fast food, Tom's gut flora consisted of approximately 3,500 species of bacteria. On the McDonald's diet, he lost 1,300 of them.[24] That's *37 percent* of his beneficial microbes killed off in less than ten days! Considering that our immunity is based not only on the strength of our friendly bacteria but on their diversity as well, that is really bad news for fast food junkies.*

SODA

Thankfully, I can't even remember the last time I had a soda; it's probably been six or seven years. I stopped cold turkey when I was in the middle of my weight loss journey and saw a poster that showed the sixteen teaspoons of sugar (probably high-fructose corn syrup, actually) in the average twenty-ounce bottle of soda. That just seemed crazy! And it occurred to me that, by getting rid of soda alone, it would be easier to lose weight.

And soda is more than sugar. Loaded with caffeine, artificial colors and flavors, and other chemicals, soda is a cheap and easy way to gain weight, generate mood swings, kill your critters, and generally harm your health. But that hasn't stopped us; Americans drink an average of forty-one gallons of soda per year. And that's just an *average*, so for every one of me—who doesn't drink any—there's someone guzzling over eighty gallons per year or more!

But it's not all bad news. Our soda consumption has gone down in the last ten years from an average of 53 gallons,[25] and water has taken back the crown as the most consumed beverage in the country. We are waking up!

---

* If you want to learn more about fast foods and how they affect the body, watch the documentary *Super Size Me* (Sony Pictures, 2004), directed by Morgan Spurlock. He eats food from McDonald's exclusively for thirty days and the results are jaw-dropping.

More Bad News about Processed Foods

THEY'RE ADDICTIVE:[26] Oh boy, it seems like all the stuff you love is addictive . . . but in this department, processed foods go beyond sugar and dairy. You see, processed foods have been *designed* to get you hooked. Through careful research, testing, and tweaking in scientific labs, food companies have created products specifically geared to hit your "bliss point" when you eat them. My Cheetos were a perfect example—the way they sort of *dissolved* in my mouth fooled my body into thinking that they weren't overly caloric. All these tricks are totally intentional on the part of industrial food corporations, and your mouth is their target. Once they've hit it, they will go to great lengths to keep you as a customer, even discrediting scientific studies that show that their products are doing you harm.[27]

Sound familiar? Well, guess who owns—or has owned—some of the biggest food companies on earth? The tobacco companies! Who knows better how to create and manipulate addicts?

START WHERE YOU ARE: Don't let all this bad news freak you out. Every journey starts with the first step. So, if you're currently eating five fast food meals a week, go down to four. Then three . . . and so on. This is not a competition or about being perfect; it's about realizing the power of your body. By reducing extreme foods and reaching for the healing ones, your body will gets tons of feedback about how food is affecting it, and slowly but surely, its wisdom will take back the steering wheel. *Your* job is to be willing to make little shifts, and to listen to what your body is telling you.

Factory-Farmed Meat

What do I mean by factory-farmed?

In the United States, 99 percent of chickens, 94 percent of pigs, and 78 percent of cattle are raised on what we call "factory" farms.* These are large, industrial operations that house thousands of animals. The Environmental Protection Agency refers to them as AFOs, which stands for Animal Feeding Operations. Even bigger AFOs are called CAFOs, which means Concentrated Animal Feeding Operations. These are enormous outfits, designed to feed a lot of Americans.

So what's the problem?

---

* Recently, farmed fish overtook their wild brethren as our chief source of fish.

THE POWER OF FOOD

First of all, factory farms are stinky, toxic, and overcrowded hellholes, terrible not just for the animals, but for our environment as well.[28] The manure produced on factory farms alone is a huge problem, as the animals create much more fecal matter than humans do, without flushing toilets and water treatment plants. This CAFO poop, which includes antibiotics, hormones, and deadly bacteria like E. coli, has been known to spill, overflow, and even seep into local water tables.[29] It's a crappy situation (yes, I went there).

Beyond the excrement, CAFOs are the furthest thing from natural. Animals live in overcrowded, putrid, unsanitary conditions[30] and are fed—or injected with—things that are completely foreign to their bodies. Hey, I eat animals, but I don't believe they should be treated badly. Americans are rediscovering more natural and ethical ways of raising livestock.

By the way, you won't see "factory-farmed" or "CAFO" stamped onto these meats. No one wants to remind you of where they come from. But you will see "organic," "grass-fed," "antibiotic-free," or "hormone-free" labels on meat products that are better quality. Buy those.

Let's take a look at factory-farmed meat using our Three Concepts:

1.   *Is factory-farmed meat whole?*

It depends. Meat is a whole food. However, processed meats (hot dogs, tinned meat, many cold cuts, etc.) are not whole, and are often treated with chemicals and added sugar.

2.   *Do factory-farmed meats cause inflammation?*

Yes. You see, factory-farmed animals are fed crappy food. Cows are meant to eat wild grasses, but those raised on factory farms primarily eat grains (like corn) or soybeans, along with just about any other cheap "food" their owners can get away with.[31]* This might include sawdust,[32] leftover baked goods,[33] and even stranger stuff; I saw a CNN report on a farmer who fed his cattle candy![34]

Just like you have a whole and perfect body, so does a cow, and when it is fed extreme foods that don't support its body's functions, it suffers. So a diet of grains (for which a cow's body is not designed) upsets the balance of fats in its body, specifically skewing its ratio of omega-6 to omega-3 fatty acids, which lead directly to . . . inflammation, in the animal and in those who eat its meat.

Not good.

Also, the corn (or soy) fed to factory-farmed animals is genetically modified, just like the roughly 90 percent of the corn and soybeans grown in the United States—it's a cheap way to produce a lot of food.[35] That means that the cow's lunch has withstood a *ridiculous* amount of toxic herbicides.[36] See the sidebar on GMOs to learn more.

---

* Believe it or not, even some farmed fish are routinely fed corn and soy, too!

Where do those toxins go after they've entered the animal? Well, some are simply excreted, while others are valiantly processed by the liver. But many of these toxins end up going to the animal's brain and fat deposits. So the average factory-farmed cow or pig is chock-full of environmental toxins,[37] which are big drivers of inflammation. And when we humans eat the meat from these antibiotic-treated, unhealthy, and generally bummed-out animals, we take all of that rough stuff in, too. According to nutrition researcher T. Colin Campbell, 90 to 95 percent of our exposure to environmental chemicals comes from eating meat and dairy.[38] And don't think that cutting the fat off a steak will help; most of the fat is marbled into the meat.

So yeah, factory-farmed meat is really not good.

WHY SO MUCH CORN?

Corn seems to be everywhere. It's in practically every processed food; we feed it to our livestock; we refine it into high-fructose corn syrup, and we even add it to our gasoline, in the form of ethanol! Why, oh why, is there so much corn? Good question.

Well, since the 1930s, the U.S. government has offered financial help to farmers in the form of subsidies. This is generally a good thing because farming is a risky proposition: While one year's crops are bountiful, others are meager. With financial support, farmers are less vulnerable to the weather, pests, and fluctuating markets. Subsidies help the whole food system to remain relatively stable in the face of Nature's unknowns, but they also encourage farmers (who take the form of big corporations as well as small, family-owned farms these days) to grow the subsidized crops, which can lead to big surpluses. And the crops that are most subsidized? Corn, wheat, soybeans, rice, and cotton. So, thanks to government subsidies, we now have lots and *lots* of cheap, genetically modified corn. So cheap, in fact, that we have found ways to put it, as a filler, sweetener, or additive, into just about everything. Frito, anyone?

3. *Is factory-farmed meat good for gut bacteria?*

You gotta be kidding me.

Here is where it goes from bad to worse. Factory-farmed animals are routinely given antibiotics . . . and not just here and there. In 2012, almost fifteen million kilograms of antibiotics were sold for use on animals in the United States,[39] while humans were given just over three million kilograms.[40] That's 77 percent of all antibiotics in this country being used on animals, mostly livestock. And it's not simply because they are standing around in their own poop, crammed shoulder-to-shoulder, getting sick—although that's a factor. Antibiotics promote growth in the animals, so American farmers get more bang for their buck if a cow, or a pig, or a chicken is pumped up on these pharmaceuticals.* Even fish farmed in the United States are given antibiotics to prevent disease and grow faster.[41]

But this leads to two enormous problems. First, it means that when you eat conventional meat, you may ingesting antibiotic residue. In 2012, the Food and Drug Administration issued seventy-eight warning letters to livestock producers whose meat samples "bore traces of illegal drugs or of residues that were illegally high."[42] As we discussed, antibiotics wipe out your critters, which is great if you have a serious infection but *not* so great if you don't. So by eating factory-farmed meat, you are weakening your immunity.

The second scary problem is even scarier: The overuse of antibiotics—on humans and on livestock—is causing nasty bacteria to get *stronger*. It turns out that unfriendly bacteria are constantly adapting and evolving to get around our antibiotic barriers, forcing us to continually develop new antibiotics to outsmart them. But we're not keeping up. Strains of what are now called "superbugs" are being discovered every day; they are ridiculously strong and resistant to our current drugs. Not only are they showing up in meats sold over the counter,[43] they also hide out in hospitals, where dose after dose of antibiotics often prove useless against them. This means people are dying, in hospitals, of infections they picked up *in the hospitals*. The Centers for Disease Control and Prevention estimates that two million people in the United States are infected with drug-resistant bacteria each year and that 23,000 of them die as a result. It's not pretty. And it all began with our overzealous use of these miracle drugs.

Fortunately, we are waking up, and California is leading the charge. Starting in 2018, antibiotics used on livestock in the Golden State will have to be ordered by a licensed veterinarian (currently farmers can buy them over the counter) and the use of antibiotics to fatten up animals will be illegal.[44] That sounds like a good start, and hopefully, the rest of the country will follow suit.

There has been some movement in the livestock industry, too. Some farmers have stopped using antibiotics prescribed for humans on their animals. Instead, they use what are called *ionophores*, which are antibiotics designed for animals only. This is meant to reduce the threat of superbugs developing strength against *our* drugs. That's progress, I suppose.

Perhaps most surprisingly, in 2015, the Perdue company began promising "No Antibiotics Ever" on its Harvestland and Simply Smart brands of chicken products, which contain neither antibiotics nor ionophores.[45] As the third-largest producer of broiler chicken in the United States, Perdue is a big enterprise, and its decision should have a wide-reaching impact. Thanks, Perdue!

---

* By the way, this type of "sub-therapeutic" use of antibiotics is illegal in Europe. They don't do it, and they don't import any American beef because of it.

GMOS: GMO stands for Genetically Modified Organism. These organisms are plants or other foods that have had genes from *other* organisms injected into their DNA, to create an entirely new organism. This is not like human reproduction or even the cross-pollination that happens in Nature. And it's not even like the hybrids of plants that farmers have been making for thousands of years. GMOs don't happen spontaneously, or through active pollination. We *make* them happen, in a lab, using sophisticated technology—like "gene canons" that shoot strands of DNA into unsuspecting nuclei.

Some important facts:

1. You are most likely eating GMOs without knowing it. The U.S. Congress has refused to pass a labeling law (unlike in Europe), so GMO ingredients have been introduced—invisibly—into most processed foods containing corn or soy. Which is basically all of them.

2. Most GMOs are owned by one big company, Monsanto, which has a long and complicated history, worth a leisurely Internet search. It was originally a chemical company!

3. Monsanto has an extensive and lucrative relationship with the U.S. government, so it experiences very little federal pushback for its actions, and legislation has traditionally favored the company's needs. Altogether, Monsanto is known for some pretty nasty practices, which you may want to learn about before letting them feed your kids.

But that's the political side of things. In terms of health, there are some other questions to ask.

Are GMOs safe? Well, they have been around for only a short period of time, so that's hard to know, for sure. What we do know is that most of the genetically modified crops in the United States are corn, soy, and cotton. And the genes of these crops have been modified to be "herbicide resistant," allowing farmers to kill all the weeds around the GMO crop plant, without hurting it. Originally, this meant less poisonous stuff on our food (and cotton). That sounds good!

Not so fast.

According to *Forbes* magazine, the amount of herbicides used on GMO crops went down only during the first few years of their use (1998 to 2001). Since then, the herbicides used on crops in the United States have increased *tenfold*. Why would that happen? Well, it turns out—just like we've seen with antibiotics—you can't outsmart Mother Nature. The weeds around these GMO crops are evolving and developing resistance to the herbicides, so now we need even more to keep them at bay! Not only do farmers have to spray more of their main herbicide—glyphosate, commercially known as Roundup (also owned by Monsanto, curiously)—but they've had to introduce new and different herbicides as well to keep up the fight. This makes for a lot of toxins on our corn, soy, and cotton. And guess who eats most of the corn and soy? Cows and other livestock. And these toxins collect in their fat, which we grill up in the kitchen.

No one is entirely sure if GMOs are harming us directly. We can't really know because most of the testing is done voluntarily by the GMO companies themselves and then simply evaluated by the U.S. government. Plus, it may take quite a while for a significant body of data to be compiled on their effects. What we do know is that GMOs in the United States have increased our exposure to environmental toxins, *a lot*.

That's enough for me. I do my best to give GMOs the heave-ho.

More Bad News about Factory-Farmed Meat

FACTORY-FARMED CATTLE ARE ALSO ROUTINELY DOSED WITH HORMONES: Three of them are naturally occurring sex hormones (estradiol, progesterone, and testosterone) while others are synthetic versions created for the cattle industry.[46] As we discussed in the section on dairy, your perfect body doesn't need any extra hormones, and too many can wreak real havoc.

Processed Oils and Salt

I'm not about demonizing oil and salt, really. I just want to say: *Use good-quality ingredients in the kitchen*. If you're going to go to all the trouble to buy better foods, spend time cooking, and pay attention to your body's needs, there's no point in using crappy spices, herbs, vinegars, soy sauce, miso, and other condiments. You only need to purchase these ingredients once in a while, so buy the best: organic whenever possible, and with no unnatural additives.

You'll be using oils and salts the most, so let's start there:

By processed oils, I mean *refined* vegetable oils, like canola (also known as rapeseed), soybean, corn, sunflower, and safflower oil. These are oils that go through a very complicated process of refinement. And hopefully you remember that the more we refine a food, the harder it is on the body. These refined oils show up in processed foods all the time.

That said, I do use safflower oil in a few of my recipes; I prefer it for deep-frying because it is taste-less, with a high smoke point. Sometimes it's the only way I can achieve a certain quality in my cook-ing. I don't get twisted up about it. Most of the time I'm using unrefined oils, like my trusty olive oil.

Other (generally) unrefined oils include: avocado, walnut, coconut, sesame, and flax. Make sure to check the label to make sure they're unrefined and organic, and to store them as directed.

So let's get to our three questions:

1.   Are refined oils whole?

Nope. No oil is whole, because it's just one piece of a whole food (coconut oil, for instance, is a product of the whole coconut). But just how "unwhole" are refined oils?

Well, back in the day, you had olives or seeds and a grindstone. And maybe a donkey to crank the grindstone in a circle. That was it. What came out was pure, unfiltered oil. Not only was it delicious, it was good for you. Humans have been making unrefined oils for thousands of years.

But with modern, industrialized food production, we have been bending over backward to create highly refined oils; production now involves multiple processes, chemicals, and treatments. We thought this was a civilized way of producing oil, but we've messed with Nature too much. That gen-erally spells trouble—as you'll see when we ask this next question . . .

2.   Do refined oils cause inflammation?

Yes. This is their biggest problem. The refining throws off the delicate balance between omega-6 and omega-3 fatty acids, which leads to inflammation. When you consider that these oils are in al-most every processed food and most fast foods, and that every potato chip you've ever eaten was deep-fried in one of them, they add up to a significant, pervasive, and silent factor in chronic inflam-mation. Refined oils are a *thing*.

3.   Are refined oils good for gut bacteria?

The research on this stuff is new, but so far scientists have concluded that only *unrefined* oils are good for gut bacteria. In one study,[47] refined olive oil and butter altered those microbial populations so that they looked more like those found in obese people, whereas unrefined virgin olive oil did not.

Refined Salt

By refined salt, I mean table salt, any salt that isn't sea salt, and all the sodium that shows up in pro-cessed foods.

Is refined salt whole?

No. What we refer to as "table salt" has been refined and stripped of the seventy-five key minerals and trace elements that come in natural sea salt, such as potassium, calcium, magnesium, and sulphur. Sea salt's mineral profile is perfectly suited to the human body. Think about it: We are salty beings. Our blood is salty, our tears are salty. Our nervous system requires electrolytes, one of which is sodium. But it's not *just* sodium. It's a host of other minerals working in conjunction with sodium, as they do in sea salt.

2. *Does refined salt cause inflammation?*

Sea salt, when it contains all its minerals, tends to be anti-inflammatory. But when salt is refined, leaving nothing but sodium chloride (and some iodine, which is added to table salt in this country), things can get wonky. A dash may not be a big deal, but understand that this stripped-down form of salt (called "sodium" on packaging) is in just about every processed food on the planet. And not in small, ladylike amounts! Excess sodium has been connected to high blood pressure, kidney disease, and liver problems. And sodium increases inflammation in patients who already suffer from high blood pressure.

So it turns out that those seventy-plus minerals that we decided to remove from sea salt are supposed to be in there. Not only do our bodies know how to use them perfectly, they are vital to our health. As we've seen with carbohydrates and meat, when we mess with Mother Nature, we just end up hurting ourselves.

DO I NEED IODINE?

Iodine is a naturally occuring element—found mostly in soil—that we all need. Without enough iodine, thyroid problems can develop, and iodine deficiencies in pregnant women can cause intellectual and developmental disabilities in their babies. To combat this, in 1924 the United States started adding iodine in the form of potassium iodide to table salt and since then, these issues have lessened in frequency. So why am I suggesting that you switch from table salt to sea salt? Does sea salt have enough iodine to prevent these problems? Well, it contains trace amounts, but the consensus is that it doesn't have as much as iodized table salt, and probably not enough for an adult. That's the bad news. The good news is that sea vegetables contain lots of iodine (kelp, hijiki, arame, and wakame all have plenty), making them the best food source of iodine there is. So as long as you're getting your seaweed on a regular basis, you should be fine.

3.   Is refined salt good for gut bacteria?

There hasn't been a ton of research on this, but it seems that too much salt of any kind is hard on your critters. A 2014 study done on mice by the American Heart Association showed that a high-salt diet altered gut bacteria significantly compared to a normal-salt diet, and reflected a composition that has recently been showing up in obesity studies.[48]

Keep in mind that sea salt is a natural preservative, so it's antibacterial. That means it will keep the bad guys at bay, but it can also depress your good ones. Moderation is key.

Phew!!!

Well done. You've just learned a *ton*. Some of it might have gone in one ear and out the other; that's okay. You have your perfect, whole body for a lifetime, and you will learn more and more as you go along. Please revisit this "Power of Food" chapter when you need inspiration or are ready to absorb more information. It will always be here for you.

Next, we get personal . . .

Let's Take a Selfie:

A Health Test

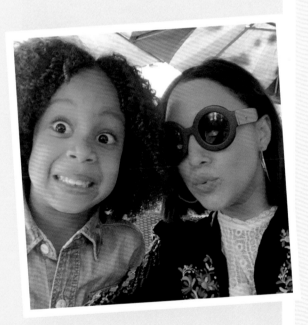

ENOUGH WITH ALL THE BIG IDEAS! IT'S time to engage with this book in an intimate way, and let it guide you on a real journey. So let's get down to the nitty-gritty. Let's talk about *you*.

Before you begin on this path to well-being, we need to know where you're at now, and in order to do that, you're going to take a selfie. But this is not the kind of selfie you put on Instagram. This one will be a picture of your current health and how it manifests in different ways: your energy, sleep, digestion, eating habits, etc. By answering the questions on the following pages, you will be making a little sketch of your life, physically, emotionally, and in terms of your goals.

This will be the BEFORE picture that you need in order to chart your progress. You can fill out this questionnaire again after doing a wake-up call, and get your first AFTER picture. The more you apply the principles you're learning, and the more you eat good food, the more changes you will see.

Since we're talking selfies, you can take an actual photograph, too, if you like!

Before you fill out this questionnaire, I recommend that you scan it into your computer. You can then download fresh copies and fill them out after your first wake-up call, after a month, or even a year from now. You'll be amazed at how much you change!

The Physical Stuff

Energy level

SCALE OF 1 TO 5 • (1 IS POOR, 5 IS FULLY ENERGIZED)

MORNING:	1	2	3	4	5
AFTERNOON:	1	2	3	4	5
EVENING:	1	2	3	4	5

Do you have enough energy to complete all your daily activities or do you feel overwhelmed?

I'VE GOT PLENTY OF ENERGY	OVERWHELMED	IT DEPENDS ON THE DAY

Sleep

Do you fall asleep easily, or toss and turn for a while?

FALLING ASLEEP IS EASY PEASY	IT TAKES ME FOREVER	IT CHANGES

How is the quality of your sleep? Scale of 1 to 5 (1 is poor, 5 is deep and restful)

1	2	3	4	5

How many hours do you sleep? __ During the week? __ On the weekend? __

Digestion

How often do you experience heartburn?

OFTEN, IT'S AN ISSUE	SOMETIMES	RARELY

Bad gas?

OFTEN, IT'S EMBARRASSING	HERE AND THERE	RARELY

Digestive pain?

OUCH! AFTER EVERY MEAL	SOMETIMES	RARELY

Constipation?

I AM REGULARLY IRREGULAR	SOMETIMES	RARELY

Diarrhea?

I'M A LOOSE CANNON	SOMETIMES	RARELY

Elimination

How often do you have bowel movements?

MORE THAN ONCE A DAY	DAILY	EVERY OTHER DAY	I HAVE NO IDEA

Are your bowel movements fast and easy or slow and difficult?

FAST AND EASY	SLOW AND DIFFICULT	DEPENDS ON THE DAY

What is the quality of your poop?

LOOSE	LONG BANANAS	SMALL, HARD BALLS

Possible alarm bells

Do you ever get headaches?

VERY RARELY	SOMETIMES	OFTEN

Any skin conditions?	YES	NO

If so, what and where on your body?

Any aches and pains?		YES	NO

If so, where and how often?

Do you get menstrual cramps?		YES	NO

IF SO, ARE THEY . . .		
SEVERE	MODERATE	MILD

Are they so bad that you take medication for them?	YES	NO

Do you experience noticeable PMS?	YES	NO

If so, how many days before your period does it start?

What are the symptoms of your PMS?

What is your current weight?

What kinds of exercise do you engage in?

How often?

Do you enjoy it?	YES	NO

Your food life

What is your current diet composed of?

AVERAGE BREAKFAST:

AVERAGE LUNCH:

AVERAGE DINNER:

AVERAGE SNACK:

If you don't have consistent meals, describe your food routine:

How do you eat?		
SITTING, WITH MUSIC AND A CANDLE	SITTING, WATCHING TV OR CHECKING EMAIL	STANDING, IN THE CAR, OR ON THE RUN

How many times would you estimate you chew an average mouthful of food?		
LESS THAN 5 CHEWS/CHOMPS	5–20 CHEWS/CHOMPS	20–50 CHEWS/CHOMPS

Favorite foods

Name a food you feel you can't live without:

Name a food (or food group) you really DON'T want to try:

Name a food (or food group) you're curious about trying:

How often do you cook for yourself?			
DAILY	1-5 TIMES/WEEK	A FEW TIMES A MONTH	NEVER
How do you feel about cooking:	IT'S MY PASSION	I'M OPEN TO EXPLORING	I HATE IT

Do you have a buddy you could cook with?	
YES	NO

If so, who?

The emotional stuff

How often do you feel anxiety?			
ALMOST ALL OF THE TIME	OFTEN	ONLY UNDER UNUSUAL STRESS	RARELY

How often do you cry?			
DAILY	WEEKLY	ONLY WHEN SOMETHING REALLY SAD IS HAPPEN- ING	NEVER

How often do you lose your temper?			
DAILY	WEEKLY	ONLY WHEN SOMEONE GETS IN MY FACE	NEVER

Does your day feel like a blur or do you have some moments of inner peace?		
BLUR!!!	BIT OF BOTH	I'M A BUDDHA

How do you feel about your relationships? With your significant other:			
I FOUND MY SOULMATE	I CHOSE WELL	WE NEED WORK	HE/SHE DRIVES ME NUTS

With your kids:			
LITTLE ANGELS	KIDS WILL BE KIDS	PARENTING IS CHALLENG- ING MOST OF THE TIME	I NEED A TRANQUILIZER

With your friends:			
I HAVE A GREAT POSSE	I'M SATISFIED	ROOM FOR IMPROVEMENT	WHAT FRIENDS?

How do you feel about yourself?			
I GENUINELY LOVE AND ACCEPT MYSELF	I'M OKAY	I WRESTLE WITH SELF- ACCEPTANCE REGULARLY	DON'T ASK

How do you feel about your life?			
LIFE IS BEAUTIFUL	LIFE IS GOOD	LIFE BAFFLES ME	I DON'T LIKE TO THINK ABOUT IT

Are you hungry for new experiences or does life feel exhausting and overwhelming?		
HUNGRY	BUSY BUT CURIOUS	EXHAUSTED

The big picture stuff

Are you able to accomplish your goals?			
YES, EASILY	YES, WITH SOME FRUS-TRATION	NOT OFTEN	NEVER

List five things that make you happy:

1.
2.
3.
4.
5.

Do you have a life dream, or a big vision you'd like to realize?	
YES	NO

If so, what is it?

Do you believe it's possible to accomplish it?

What actions are you taking to make it happen?

Do you have a spiritual practice?	
YES	NO
If so, how often do you practice it?	

Name three people you consider part of your support system:

1.
2.
3.

Can you call or get together with any of them over the next ten days?

Congratulations! You've just taken a good, hard look at yourself and your current condition. You're very brave to have done that. This selfie is a baseline against which you will be able to track your progress over time. Without this little snapshot of yourself, the results of changing your diet will be hard to spot. Armed with this information, you are enabling yourself to stay inspired and make big shifts. Yaaayyyy!!!

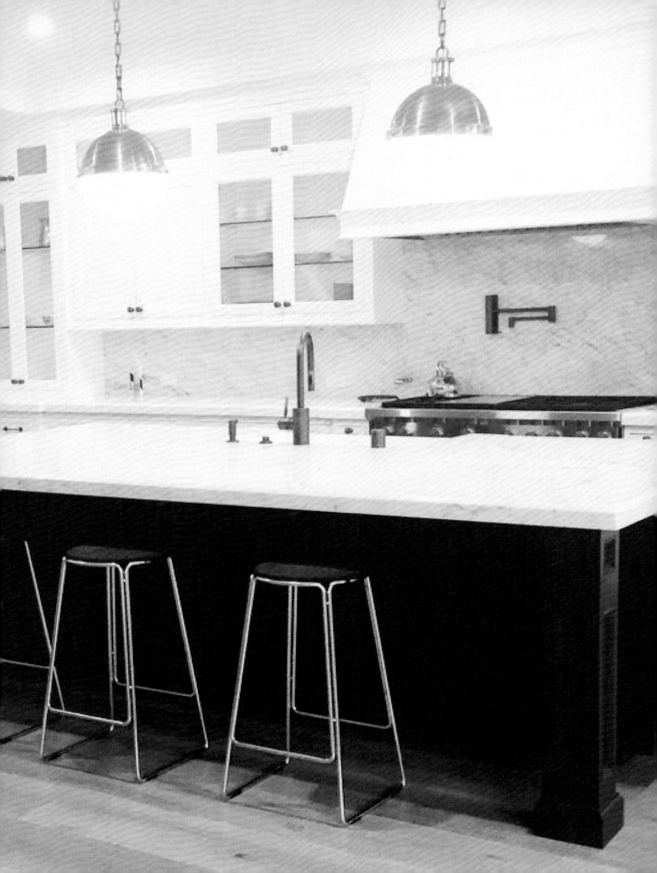

Your Wake-Up Call

I'M ABOUT TO SHOW YOU A TEN-DAY MENU plan to help kick-start your new life. It's delicious and healthy and will make you feel amazing.

However, waking up doesn't require sticking to a ten-day menu. It's not about following some complicated plan perfectly. No, no, no. Waking up is about making a commitment to start *listening to your body,* and to honor its wisdom and healing powers. And guess what? Only *you* know what that means, and only *you* know what your next step will be.

So, wake-up calls can be simple. You can do:

THE SIMPLE DROP: Drop soda for ten days and see how you feel. Or dairy. Or white sugar. Just pick one thing. Your mind will like the simplicity and hopefully enjoy the challenge. It's fun to explore all the healthy alternatives to the thing you've dropped, like fizzy fruit juice, fun dairy replacements, and safer sweets. See "Your New Pantry" on page 287 to find out what they are.

Or:

THE SIMPLE ADD: Consciously pick *up* a new food. Maybe you commit to eating fruits or vegetables at every single meal (build on my breakfast smoothie on page 243!) or a fermented food every day, or trying five types of seaweed in ten days. The Simple Add is fun because your brain won't feel deprived. It's all about more, more, MORE!

Or:

THE SWITCHEROO: This is a combination of the Drop and the Add: Drop one food that hurts and pick up one food that heals. For instance, drop white sugar and pick up . . . whole grains! Or more vegetables! For ten days. It's simple, and feels balanced.

SET YOUR GOALS: Whenever you do a wake-up call, it helps to think about the end result. Before you run a race, you imagine the finish line. If you didn't, you'd never start in the first place. And I won't lie: It's gonna be hard at times. There are going to be moments when you think about turning back, or when you're exhausted and saying, *Why am I doing this?* Written goals will help you stay the course.

Initially, I had three goals: First, I wanted to have a baby. That was incredibly important to me. Second, I wanted to be pain-free from my endometriosis. And finally, I wanted to gain control over my body, which felt totally out of whack at the time. When I focused on any of those things, they kept me going.

So what does the finish line look like for you? What are your goals? Losing weight? Getting rid of headaches? Clearing up a skin condition? Feeling happier? Reducing inflammation? Sleeping better? Focus on your goals, and they will get you there.

MY "WAKE-UP CALL" GOALS:

1.

2.

3.

4.

5.

And remember to use the selfie: I created it so you can have some information about where you are when you start. Hard data is important. Not everything is going to change in ten days, but some things *will*, and the selfie will prove that you are making progress. As time goes on and you begin to chart the deeper changes, taking more snapshots is important.

For those of you who love cooking and want to dive right in, here's your plan for the next ten days:

Ten-Day
"Wake-Me-Up"
Menu Plan

BEFORE YOU BEGIN: You will notice that this menu suggests all sorts of recipes. If you make them all, you will have a very delicious experience, believe you me. However, you don't *need* to cook that much in order to have a powerful Wake-Up Call. This is about abstaining from dairy and white sugar and eating lots of healthy food. If you don't have the time, energy, or inclination to go whole hog, just look at what each recipe is working with (a grain, a protein—meat or bean—a vegetable, or a dessert) and do your best within that category. For instance, if I suggest a slightly elaborate fish dish and you end up with a can of wild salmon seasoned with olive oil and dill, or a complicated salad leads you to steamed greens, that's *awesome*. There's no need to be tethered to the recipes. Just make sure to stick with the general theme.

When you have the time, of course, please reward yourself with a mouth-watering recipe. But the last thing I want is for you to feel pressured. Pressure rarely works over the long haul. Do what works for you, and you will succeed.

Day 1

Pssst . . . I have a confession: This ten-day plan is actually a nine-and-one-third-day plan because I begin Day 1 with an evening meal; that way, you have time to shop for ingredients during the day and get your kitchen up to speed in general. And lunches are mostly constructed from the previous dinner's leftovers, so . . . it just makes sense.

DINNER

- Salmon Croquettes (page 141)
- Ginger-Lime Roasted Rainbow Carrots (page 173)
- Kale & Almond Fried Rice (page 201)
- 1 small serving of raw unpasteurized pickle (store bought),
  or Cultured Vegetables (page 214)
- Crispy Rice Treats (page 282)

Day 2

BREAKFAST

- Large Smoothie (page 243)

LUNCH

- Leftover Salmon Croquettes mixed with mayonnaise to make a salmon salad, served in a whole wheat pita pocket
- Leftover Kale & Almond Fried Rice
- Leftover Ginger-Lime Roasted Rainbow Carrots
- Fresh salad

SNACK

- Leftover Crispy Rice Treats

DINNER

- Asparagus Soup (page 114)
- Lamb Burgers with Mint Aioli (page 121)
- Brown rice
- Dijon Roasted Cauliflower (page 174)
- Fresh salad
- 1 small serving of raw unpasteurized pickle, or cultured vegetables
- Fresh fruit

Tia Tip: **Make leftovers.** You'll see in this food plan that almost every lunch is made from the previous night's leftovers. That's because life is too damn short to be cooking all the time! I believe in cooking lots of food when I'm in the kitchen, and using the excess over the next couple of days. For instance, extra brown rice can get fried up, sauces can be drizzled here and there, and almost every vegetable can be reheated. Soups are often better the next day, and is there anything you can't roll in a tortilla? Using leftovers makes me a more creative cook and gives me more time with my family. Cook double portions and challenge yourself to repurpose the extra food.

Day 3

BREAKFAST

- Nourish Bowl (page 155)

LUNCH

- Crumbled leftover Lamb Burgers, leftover rice, and leftover cauliflower, stir-fried together with a splash of soy sauce and fresh scallions
- Fresh salad

SNACK

- Fresh fruit

DINNER

- Chickpea Burgers, naked or on whole wheat buns (page 158)
- Roasted Beet Salad (includes quinoa, page 191)
- A variety of steamed vegetables, including leafy greens
- Dark Chocolate Banana "Milk" Shake (page 270)

Day 4

BREAKFAST

- Amaranth & Millet Porridge with Bananas, Figs, & Almonds (page 233)

LUNCH

- Leftover Chickpea Burgers (either fry up yesterday's leftover burger mix, or roll into balls, like falafel, and deep-fry)
- Leftover Roasted Beet Salad
- Fresh salad

SNACK

- Leftover "Milk" Shake

DINNER

- Pan-Roasted Chicken with Maple Bacon Sauce (page 134)
- Brown rice
- Creamed Spinach (page 169)
- Steamed kale
- 1 small serving of raw unpasteurized pickle, or cultured vegetables
- Fresh fruit

Day 5

BREAKFAST

- Brown rice cereal (used for Crispy Rice Treats) with a non-dairy milk, fresh fruit, and brown rice syrup

LUNCH

- Leftover Pan-Roasted Chicken Thighs (get creative and shred chicken, and mix with some of the spinach and brown rice)
- Reheated creamed spinach
- Leftover brown rice
- Freshly steamed bok choy

SNACK

- Fresh fruit with maple syrup drizzle

DINNER

- Lentil "Meatloaf" & Shiitake Mushroom Gravy (page 128)
- Barley Salad (page 207)
- Slow-Roasted Grape Tomatoes (page 178)

- Crispy Collard Chips (page 194)
- Chocolate-Glazed Vanilla Doughnuts (page 268)

This menu includes a lot of sweet things, to help with your withdrawal from white sugar and other refined carbs. As time goes by, you might want to dial down the sweets to one serving per day or even less. Too many desserts, even the safer ones, can make you feel lethargic and make losing weight more difficult.

Day 6

BREAKFAST

- Spinach, Tomato, & Mushroom Omelet (page 241)

LUNCH

- Leftover Lentil "Meatloaf"
- Leftover Barley Salad
- Leftover Slow-Roasted Grape Tomatoes
- Fresh salad

SNACK

- Leftover Chocolate-Glazed Vanilla Doughnut

DINNER

- Turkey Meatballs (page 149) with Roasted Marinara Sauce (page 227) over zucchini or whole wheat noodles
- Twice-Baked Sweet Potatoes (page 185)
- Steamed kale
- 1 small serving of raw unpasteurized pickle, or cultured vegetables
- Peach Raspberry Crisp (page 274)

Day 7

BREAKFAST

- Large Smoothie (page 243)

LUNCH

- Leftover Turkey Meatballs in Roasted Marinara Sauce, reheated and served in a whole wheat pita pocket
- Reheated Twice-Baked Sweet Potatoes
- Fresh salad

SNACK

- Big bowl of Party Popcorn (page 253)

DINNER

- Fish Chowder (page 109)
- Fresh quinoa
- Ginger-Lime Roasted Rainbow Carrots (page 173)
- Steamed bok choy with Creamy Pumpkin Dressing (page 222)
- 1 small serving of raw unpasteurized pickle, or cultured vegetables
- Summer Sorbet (page 286)

Day 8

BREAKFAST

- Banana Pancakes with Blistered Blueberries (page 234)

LUNCH

- Leftover Fish Chowder over leftover quinoa
- Leftover Ginger-Lime Roasted Rainbow Carrots
- Fresh salad with leftover Pumpkin Dressing

SNACK

- Summer Sorbet

DINNER

- Miso Soup (page 213)
- Thai Beef Lettuce Cups (page 144)
- Brown rice
- Hijiki Seaweed with Onions & Carrots (page 188)
- Steamed greens
- Fresh fruit

Day 9

BREAKFAST

- Brown rice cereal with non-dairy milk (or any other cereal without white sugar or dairy)

LUNCH

- Leftover beef and leftover rice, stir-fried in sesame oil with a splash of soy sauce and seasonings to taste, served in a whole wheat pita (if desired)
- Fresh salad

SNACK

- Classic or Edamame Hummus (page 247 or 248) with raw vegetables and rice crackers

DINNER

- Butternut Squash Soup (page 105)
- Quinoa

- Shrimp and Broccoli Ginger Stir-Fry (page 142)
- Steamed greens
- 1 small serving of raw unpasteurized pickle, or cultured vegetables
- No-Churn Chocolate Espresso Ice Cream (page 267)

Day 10

BREAKFAST

- Amaranth & Millet Porridge with Bananas, Figs, & Almonds (page 233)

LUNCH

- Leftover Butternut Squash Soup
- Leftover quinoa
- Leftover Shrimp and Broccoli Ginger Stir-Fry
- Fresh salad

SNACK

- Leftover No-Churn Chocolate Espresso Ice Cream

DINNER

- Chicken Noodle Soup (page 102)
- Grilled "Cheese" Sandwich (page 254)
- 1 small serving of raw unpasteurized pickle, or cultured vegetables
- Steamed Napa cabbage and other vegetables
- Fresh fruit

What to Expect
from a Wake-Up Call

Everyone's different, so it's impossible to predict exactly what you'll experience over the next ten days. However, sugar and dairy are powerful foods, and I thought it might be useful to list some of the reactions common among those who let them go and eat more natural foods.

When you let go of white sugar and other highly refined carbs, you may experience:

- Sadness
- Fatigue
- Anger
- Cravings
- Night Sweats
- Crying
- Anxiety
- Headaches

What to do during the wake-up call:

- Eat lots of safer sweets
- Chew food well
- Journal
- Call a friend and have a weep!

What to expect by the end:

- More balanced energy
- Emotional peace
- Freedom from cravings
- Better sleep
- Feeling cooler in your body
- More emotional detachment from all foods
- Weight loss
- Freedom from vending machines!!!

When you let go of dairy you may experience:

- Coughing up phlegm or other types of mucus discharge
- Acne or other skin issues
- Moodiness

- Brain fog
- Bloating
- Headaches
- Mild cravings

What to do during the wake-up call:
- Eat dairy alternatives
- Get enough fat to feel satisfied

What to expect at the end:
- Mental clarity
- Weight loss
- Feeling lighter in your body
- Feeling cooler in your body
- Clearer skin
- Detachment from dairy cravings

SETBACKS

Did I say setbacks? I meant *learning experiences!*

Let's face it: Very few of us are perfect about this stuff. It's a rare person who starts a whole new life regimen and never wavers.

Luckily, you live in a learning machine: your body. So when you kick dairy for ten days and then spread cream cheese on your bagel, your intestines will talk to you about it. When you skip sugar for a month and then dunk your head under the chocolate fountain at your cousin's wedding, it's not gonna go unnoticed by your pancreas. Or your drama-filled dreams that night.

So relax in the understanding that your brain doesn't have to be on guard 24/7. If you slip—*when* you slip—your body will let you know. Your job is to listen, and learn. Without judgment. Judging yourself will just make you neurotic.

One of the best ways to learn, even through setbacks, is to journal about the new and different things you feel. Maybe after two days, you feel exhausted, but after seven, you feel amazing! When you record your journey, you are more likely to stick to it and learn from it.

Like anything else, it's a process: As you feed your body whole foods, and really pay attention when you *don't,* it will eventually take back the steering wheel.

Doing It

IN THIS CHAPTER, WE'LL GO OVER THE practical aspects of eating and living in a more wholesome way. Let's start with the basics:

Making a Meal

What does the average meal look like?

Great question. Without getting crazy about it, think of a healthy lunch or dinner as including roughly the following:

THREE parts VEGETABLES: And yes, that's a lot of vegetables! They can be sautéed, baked, roasted, puréed, fermented, in soups, in salads, or simply eaten raw. But a healthy meal includes lots and lots of vegetables. Make sure a lot of them are green, and a small portion of them should be sea vegetables (two to three small servings per week).

ONE part WHOLE GRAINS: Brown rice, quinoa, millet, buckwheat, barley, or another grain. Best if eaten whole. Eat whole-grain products (breads and noodles) here and there, roughly three times per week.

ONE part PROTEIN: Either animal protein (organic beef, poultry, fish, or eggs) or plant-based protein (beans or bean products). Listen to your body, and not that voice that says, "You need more *protein*!" That's not your body talking; that's our society.

PLUS: Cultured vegetables: Eat at least one tablespoon of cultured vegetables or unpasteurized pickles per day. But don't go crazy with them; fermented foods can deliver a lot of salt, and it's easy to go overboard.

PLUS: Fruits, safer sweets, and desserts. These show up on a regular basis to make life sweet and enjoyable, but they are not the center of your diet. They are *treats*.

Breakfasts break the rules a little more. Fewer vegetables, maybe more grain . . . more fruit . . . it's up to you.

So that's pretty easy: 3-1-1-Plus-Plus. I smell a catchy tagline: "Dial 3-1-1-Plus-Plus for a New You!!!" I know, I know. Needs some work.

By the way, I understand that you're not going to do this perfectly. I get that sometimes lunch is a slice of Chocolate Cake (page 277). But when you eat a meal that includes vegetables, whole grains, and good-quality protein, in the ratio I suggest, you will feel fantastic and your body will thank you. It is a healthy and a satisfying way to live.

Shop to Succeed

On page 287 at the back of the book, I have included a section called "Your New Pantry." It includes all sorts of foods and products that can replace what you currently use. You'll be happy to see that every type of dairy product now has a delicious non-dairy substitute; with safer treats, life can continue to be sweet. It's important that you have lots of delicious, healthy choices, and that you know how to find them. Without these alternatives, you may be setting yourself up to fail—so check them out!

Planning

STOCK UP: I always have the staple ingredients—like dried goods, olive oil, sea salt, pepper, and garlic—on hand. If I always have them handy, I can cook something amazing with whatever fresh ingredients I buy. And the great thing about most of these staples is that they last; you don't need to buy new garlic every week. Or onions. Or whole grains. They last a while.

CHOP AHEAD: Over the weekend, or at the beginning of the week, I put on some Beyoncé and chop up some of the essentials that I use in my favorite dishes—especially the heartier ones, like onions, carrots, and celery. You can also buy them pre-chopped, at some stores. This can save a lot of time during cooking, so think through the meals you want and figure out what you can do ahead of time, without compromising freshness.

THINK IT THROUGH: I have a friend who has a whiteboard right in her kitchen. Every week, she writes down what she's going to cook for the next seven days. It's fantastic! She'll have Taco Tuesday, or Spaghetti Wednesday, etc. That way, she and her kids are always aware of what's coming and she can plan—and create—accordingly.

Feeding Kids

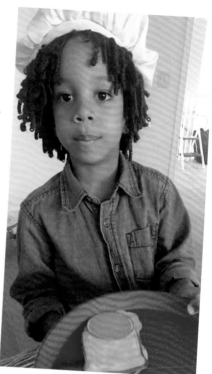

Speaking of kids, the key to feeding them healthy food is perspective, and you can only get that through experience. For a while, Cory and I let Cree eat whatever he wanted. So of course, he went for some not-so-healthy foods. Then he started to complain about his back, and his stomach. We went to the doctor, who ordered an X-ray. It turned out Cree was soooo backed up, the poor thing was in pain.

It was a real lesson to us all, and that's what I mean by perspective; feeding kids healthy food can feel like a virtuous ideal or a nightly tug-of-war, when in reality it's immensely powerful and practical. Less complaining! Less fear! Fewer visits to the doctor! When I finally got that perspective on what the bad foods do to my child, I made feeding him well a priority.

Tips for Feeding Kids Good Foods

In many ways, kids are just like adults; sometimes they're in the mood for fruits and veggies, and sometimes they're not. When I feel like Cree isn't getting enough healthy, fresh food, I do the following:

- I make smoothies: I throw in watermelon, strawberries, pineapple, and even a little avocado, broccoli, and/or spinach. He doesn't notice! And all the while, he's getting fiber, vitamins, and minerals. Go Mommy!
- I throw tons of vegetables—and even sea vegetables, like wakame—

into a soup, then purée it and season it well. To Cree, it's just a savory soup! To me, it's a godsend.

- Meatballs, anyone? I love putting spinach and other vegetables into meat dishes, like meatballs, burger, or meatloaf. They go down nice and easy.
- I serve not-so-sexy vegetables with foods I know Cree enjoys already. For example, I'll serve chicken teriyaki with some Brussels sprouts on the side. Eating a vegetable is not such a big deal when he's already happy, eating one of his favorite dishes.
- I keep things separate. Kids are funny in this department, and I find that Cree doesn't like things mixed together. So I put vegetables out separately, with a sweet or savory sauce on the side. That way he can dip his own food, and he gets a grown-up sense of control.

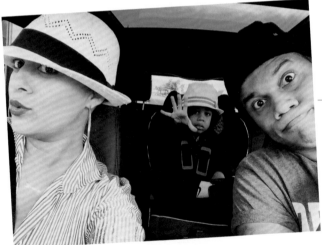

Travel

How you handle travel depends on your needs. When I was healing from endometriosis and wanted nothing more than to get pregnant, I packed my food and brought it with me everywhere, even on trips. I went to great lengths to make sure I stuck to my Body Ecology diet regimen. Since then, I've loosened up somewhat, but now I want to eat well on the road because I want to *feel* well on the road. That's really important to me. So I do the following:

PRE-TRAVEL HOMEWORK: With the Internet, there are no excuses anymore! It's easy with apps like Yelp to figure out what's in, or near, the place I'm going. I aim for Whole Foods Market or health-food stores in the area. That way, I can pick up enough of their cooked foods for a couple of days at a time. I also comb the local restaurants to find out which ones have good-quality ingredients and good reviews. It's never been so easy to get information before traveling.

PACK SOME THINGS: Sometimes it's helpful to bring a few things along for the ride. Not only are green teabags, stevia, and a ziplock bag of granola or nuts lifesavers in emergency hunger situations, they also serve as a simple reminder that I *care* about what goes in my body. Obviously, I can't live on those things, but they help me stay in my self-care gear in a world that beckons me to eat a cheeseburger.

EATING OUT: When ordering at a restaurant, I do my best to stay away from dairy and white sugar. Both make me feel crappy, and that's the last thing I want on a trip away from home. You'd be amazed how many restaurants have items that fulfill these requirements, and when in doubt, I'm not afraid to specify: "Skip the Parmesan," "No sauce, thanks," or "Can I get those steamed?" Asking for what you need is a muscle; if yours needs a workout, go for it. Restaurants should want to make customers happy.

Better restaurants may also serve meat that is organic, grass-fed, and antibiotic-free. If it doesn't say so on the menu, the meat is probably from a factory farm—so go meatless for that meal.

ONE MORE THING ABOUT TRAVEL: Sometimes being on the road feels like a wonderful excuse to break all the rules and toss commitment to the wind. That's the best thing about traveling to new places, and seeing new things—it's liberating.

But when I was healing, I couldn't afford that "freedom." And I had to really question whether loosening my boundaries was *truly* a type of freedom. I realize now that my ability to have my son was real freedom. My stable moods, nonstop energy, and the belly laughs I share at work are the freedoms I care about most—freedom from emotional pain, lethargy, and self-centered worry. And they all come from how I eat, and my commitment to that way of eating. Scarfing down pizzas in Italy may feel liberating, but it's a momentary release, often followed by a cheese hangover and remorse. That's not real freedom.

If you have tips on travel, feeding kids, or any other practical suggestions, please share them with all of us on Instagram or Twitter.

Eating around the world: If you plan to travel outside the United States, you may be in luck. Besides the Arctic, where food may be spare, traditional foods in many countries are abundant and quite healthy—it's really here in North America that we're confronted with fast food at every turn! If you look beyond the cheese in Italian cuisine, you'll find a dazzling array of fresh vegetables, whole grains, and wild fish that will make you feel *fantastico*. Skip the cream in France, and you'll find lovely salads, delicate veggies (haricots verts, anyone?), and good-quality meats (the European Union has banned growth hormones and unnecessary antibiotics in livestock). Many other European countries also prioritize whole, fresh, and local foods. In South America, there are lots of local dishes made from whole grains, beans, and vegetables, while in Asia, rice, veggies, fish, and even pickles dominate the menu. Meanwhile, in most African countries, fast food restaurants are so few and far between that fresh, local foods are still the norm. Bon voyage!

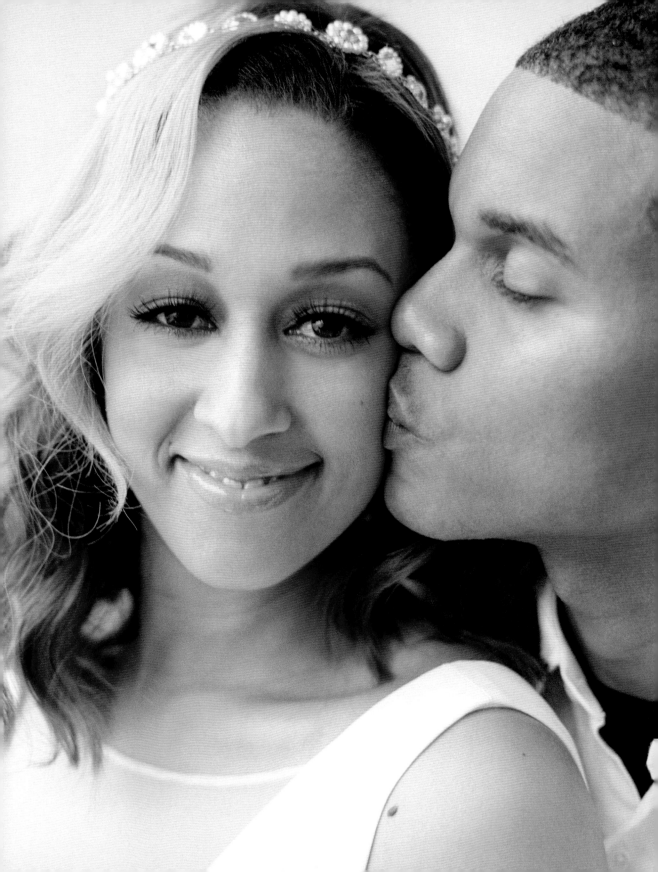

Your Whole New Life

WHEN I STARTED TO EAT DIFFERENTLY, I started to *live* differently. It was exciting. It was as if the food that was making my body stronger and healthier was having a ripple effect, and I began to make better choices across the board. Let's look at how eating better food might change your life, on both a practical and a spiritual level.

Yoga

These days, it seems like there's a yoga place on every corner of every big city. It's very popular. You may be an accomplished yogini already!

I love yoga, but for me, it's important that I'm doing it for the sanity as opposed to the vanity. It's easy to approach yoga as nothing but a workout. But really, yoga is about balancing mind, body, and spirit. That's the kind of yoga I practice. A good yoga class feels like a therapy session. I leave a lot of emotional crap on the mat. Sometimes I cry. I try to release tension—and even a few layers of my ego—in the studio, so I can emerge a better person.

And it's important to remember that yoga's not a competition. It's not about looking at myself, or trying to be perfect. It's not about outstretching that woman in the corner with the panda tattoo. I've tried that, and it undermines my whole experience. In fact, these days I won't even go to a yoga studio with mirrors on the walls! If I can't do a pose 100 percent properly, who cares? Yoga is about connecting with myself and finding a soft, generous balance—inside and out. Back in the day, the original yogis were really wise; they knew that it was all connected. They *got* it.

Acupuncture

If you've never tried acupuncture, it may sound strange—and even a little scary. But this form of Chinese medicine has been practiced for at least 2,000 years, and some believe it's been more like 4,000.

Acupuncture views the body as a whole, with every system connected and affecting all the others. Through careful observation and subtle pulse and tongue diagnosis, the acupuncturist determines where your overall energy is blocked, weak, or wonky. By inserting hair-thin needles (you can hardly feel them, I promise!) into points along energy meridians, or pathways, on the body, the acupuncturist nudges it to release stagnation and rebalance itself.

I just love acupuncture because it feels like a deep, natural medicine. It looks at the underlying causes of symptoms, not just the symptoms themselves. Sure, Western medicine has its strengths—and often achieves miraculous feats—but it tends to focus exclusively on illness, crisis, and the body's bits and pieces.

Eastern medicine is more focused on and strives to support overall wellness. Acupuncturists respect that the body is whole and—left to its own devices—works perfectly. I like that. Whenever I'm feeling run-down, or want to shift something in my body, I go to acupuncture.

One more thing: Most acupuncturists also have an incredibly sophisticated knowledge of healing plants and herbs. It takes at least four years to become proficient in traditional Chinese medicine—it's no joke. So after a treatment, you might get sent home with some healing tea that smells like bark. I prefer that to a pill, any day.

Finally, many insurance companies will cover acupuncture these days, so check it out!

Spiritual Stuff

I've always had faith, but when I started eating whole foods, it got stronger. I realized that when I took care of my body, I was supporting my spirit, too. Of course, I'm not here to talk about specific religions or spiritual paths, but I want to issue a happy warning: By eating natural foods, you will feel connected—to yourself, to others, and to Nature's bigger picture.

You are what you eat. We've talked about that quite a bit. And when you bypass the drive-through, or the factory, or the soda machine, and eat straight from Nature's cupboard, you will change, in amazing and wonderful ways. Big puzzle pieces fall into place, because it's all connected. When you start taking care of your body, your mind will be healthier as well—and when you're looking after both, you feel pulled to take care of your spirit. And that will make you a happier person who is nicer to other people, because when you love yourself you can truly love others.

I never knew that until I started doing it. It took a scary visit to the doctor and a shocking diagnosis for me to discover the power of food—to learn the secret that whole foods make *us* whole, on every level. But there's nothing stopping you from experiencing these truths right now.

Finally

If you haven't already, it's time to stop the reading and start the cooking. Ideas are powerful, but whole foods will literally change your health. And your future.

I can describe—in many ways—what I think you will experience, what to expect from this journey, and how you will feel . . . but these predictions don't really matter. The next shift is going to take place in your kitchen. And in your body. It's time to pick up that wooden spoon and stir up your life.

Thank you so much for taking this ride with me, and for giving me the chance to pass on what I've been so lucky to learn. Writing this book has been a great pleasure and privilege. It's powerful stuff. So . . .

You go, girl!

XO, Lia

RECIPES

Soups

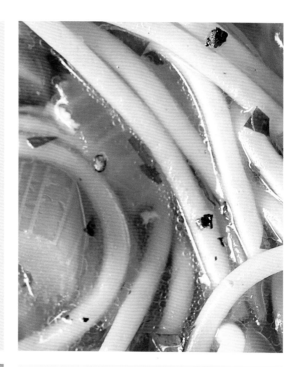

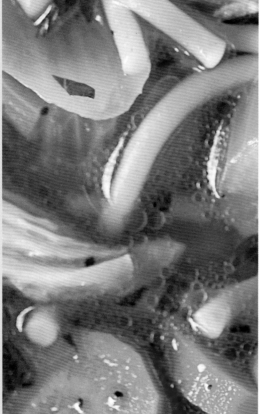

Soup is a lovely way to start a meal; it forces us to slow down, relaxes the digestive organs, and opens us up for nourishment. In this section, I've included a wide variety of soups—from chilled watermelon to chunky chili— so you can get a sense of the endless possibilities. Enjoy!

What do I need?

You don't need much to get started. Here is a list of the bare essentials to get you up and running in the kitchen:

- One or two good sharp knives
- Cutting board (I like wood or bamboo)
- Mixing bowls
- Saucepans (pots) of different sizes
- Heavy pot with a heavy lid (for cooking grains)
- Decent skillet or frying pan
- Wooden spoons
- Spatula
- Food processor, blender, or immersion blender
- Baking sheets

These items will get you started on the simpler recipes. You can expand your collection of tools as you tackle the more complicated ones. Here is a list of the equipment I use in this book (you may very well have some or all of it):

- Slow cooker
- Deep-fry thermometer
- Roasting pan
- Wok or deep skillet
- Cast iron skillet

- Nonstick skillet
- Loaf pan
- Pizza pan
- 4-quart Dutch oven
- Waffle iron
- Muffin tins
- Cooling rack
- Steamer basket
- Parchment paper
- Sieves and strainers
- Spiralizer
- Potato masher
- Grater
- Whisk
- Vegetable peeler
- Glass or stainless steel airtight containers for cultured vegetables (Mason jars, or flip-lid jars)
- Food-safe rubber gloves (for making kimchi)

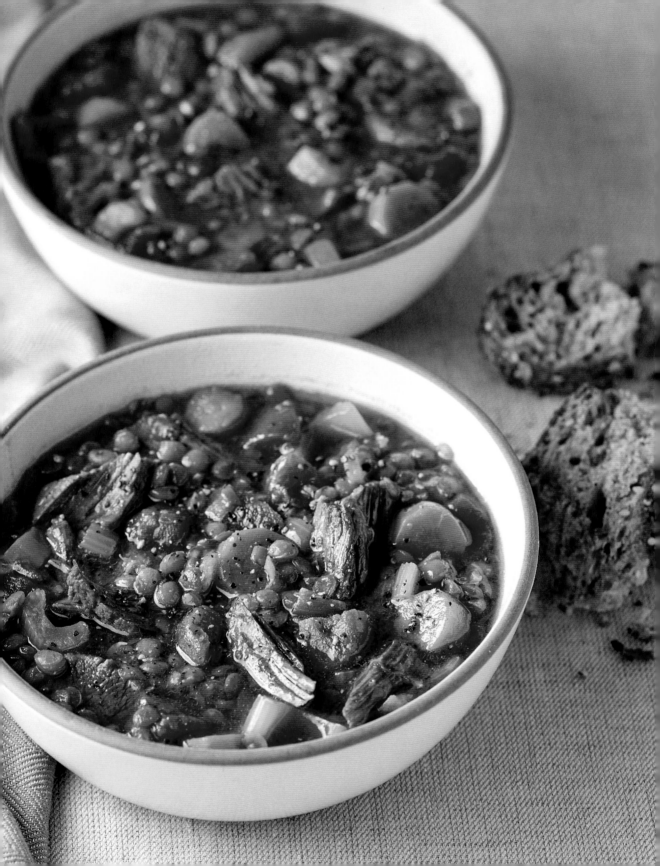

BEEF & LENTIL SOUP

g-f*

clean

Lentils are crazy good for you. They are high in protein, fiber, complex carbs, and even minerals. Combine them with beef and this is a powerhouse dish, great for family and entertaining. Because it's cooked slowly, it's very satisfying and nourishing.

Serves 8

2	celery stalks, chopped
2	carrots, sliced into 1/2-inch-thick coins
1	large yellow onion, chopped
2	garlic cloves, smashed
1	14.5-ounce can diced tomatoes
1	dried bay leaf
2-inch	sprig of fresh rosemary
1	teaspoon sea salt (plus more to taste)
	Freshly ground black pepper to taste
2	tablespoons soy sauce or tamari
1	tablespoon Dijon mustard
4	cups beef broth
1	cup brown lentils
1 1/2	pounds beef chuck, cut into 1-inch cubes
	Non-Dairy Parmesan "Cheese" to garnish (optional) (recipe on page 229)

1. Add the celery, carrots, onion, garlic, tomatoes, bay leaf, rosemary, salt, pepper, soy sauce (or tamari), mustard, and broth to a slow cooker. Give it a good stir, to make sure everything is well mixed. Stir in the lentils and the beef.

2. Turn the slow cooker onto high. Let the soup cook for at least 6 hours, or until the beef is tender and falling apart and the soup has thickened up considerably. Discard the rosemary stem. Ladle into bowls to serve. Top with cheese, if desired.

* GLUTEN-FREE IF YOU USE TAMARI.

CHICKEN NOODLE SOUP

 *g-f** A classic. Chicken noodle soup warms the body and the soul.

Serves 6

8	chicken thighs
	Sea salt to taste
1	tablespoon extra-virgin olive oil
1	medium yellow onion, chopped
4	carrots, sliced into 1/4-inch-thick coins
3	stalks of celery, sliced into 1/2-inch-thick pieces
3	garlic cloves, smashed
8	cups water
	Handful of fresh flat-leaf parsley, chopped
4	ounces uncooked whole wheat spaghetti (or gluten-free noodles), broken into 2-inch pieces

1. Generously season the chicken with salt. In a 4-quart pot, heat 2 teaspoons of oil until shimmering. Add 4 pieces of chicken, skin-side down. Cook until deep golden underneath. Turn the thighs, and cook on the other side until golden. Transfer chicken to a deep dish or bowl. Repeat with the remaining pieces of chicken. (Note: The chicken is not cooked through yet; it'll finish cooking in the soup.)

2. Spoon out of pot, and discard, all but 2 teaspoons of oil the cooking of the chicken has produced. Add the onion, carrots, celery, and garlic to the pot. Season with salt. Sauté until the onions are slightly tender and golden, about 2 minutes (if the pot begins to get dry, add the remaining teaspoon of olive oil).

3. Return the chicken to the pot, pouring in any juices from the dish. Add the water and parsley to the pot. Increase heat to high. Once the soup begins to boil, reduce the heat to a simmer. Cook for 20 minutes. Add the pasta to the soup and cook for 15 to 20 minutes more, until the pasta is as tender as you like it.

continued on next page

* GLUTEN-FREE IF YOU USE GLUTEN-FREE NOODLES.

SOUPS

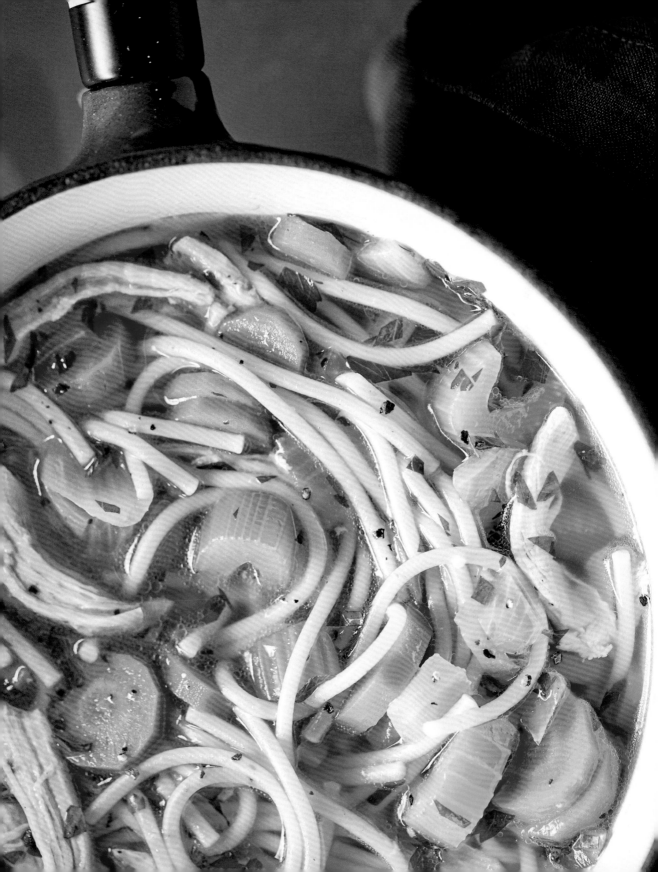

4. Remove the chicken from the pot and shred the meat from half of the chicken thighs. Save the meat from the remaining thighs to use in another recipe later in the week (it's a great add-in for the Vietnamese Rice Noodle Salad on page 205, the Kale & Almond Fried Rice on page 201, or your favorite chicken salad recipe).

5. Stir the shredded chicken into the pot. Ladle the soup into deep bowls, and serve hot.

Variation: Without the noodles, this makes a wonderful bone broth for use in other recipes.

BUTTERNUT SQUASH SOUP

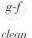

g-f

clean

This soup is easy, creamy, and great for digestion. What I love most about squash soups are that they yield a lot of satisfaction and require relatively little work in the kitchen. Small effort—big payoff!

Serves 4

2	tablespoons extra-virgin olive oil
1	head of fennel, thinly sliced (bulb only, reserve fronds for garnish)
1	large leek, chopped
	Sea salt to taste
20	ounces cubed butternut squash
3 to 4	cups vegetable broth
	Freshly grated zest of ¹/₂ an orange

1. In a 4-quart pot, heat the oil over medium heat until shimmering. Add the fennel, leek, and salt. Sauté until the fennel and leek are slightly tender, 4 to 5 minutes. Add the squash and vegetable broth. Increase heat to high and bring to a boil. Reduce heat to low. Simmer until the squash is very tender, about 20 minutes. Stir in the orange zest.

2. Working in batches, purée the soup in a blender until smooth. Ladle the soup into deep bowls. Garnish with chopped fennel fronds to serve.

How to Clean a Leek: Leeks are beautiful, elegant, delicious . . . and tricky to clean! As they grow, soil can collect between each silky leaf. Here's what to do: Slice lengthwise, starting at the bottom of the leek, keeping the root intact. You will be left with two long half-leeks with many layers of leaves. Place one half under running water, or in a big bowl of water. Carefully separate (but don't completely detach!) each leaf, exposing and rinsing off any hidden dirt. Repeat with the other half of the leek. You can then place each half-leek on a cutting board and chop it with all its newly clean leaves intact.

SLOW-COOKER BLACK BEAN SOUP

g-f

veg

clean

I love this soup, with its Mexican flair and bright flavors.

Serves 6

2	cups dried black beans
1	large onion, chopped
2	garlic cloves, chopped
1	red bell pepper, seeded and chopped
1 to 2	teaspoons sea salt
	Handful of fresh cilantro, chopped (plus more for garnish)
	Freshly ground black pepper
4	cups vegetable broth
6	tortilla chips, crumbled
1	avocado, pitted and diced
1	plum tomato, chopped
6	lime wedges

1. Add the black beans, onion, garlic, bell pepper, salt, cilantro, black pepper, and vegetable broth to a slow cooker. Cook on the low setting for 8 hours, or overnight, until the beans are very tender.

2. Transfer half of the soup to a blender. Pulse until it forms a chunky purée. Stir the purée back into the pot with the remaining soup.

3. Ladle the soup into deep serving bowls. Garnish with the tortilla chips, cilantro, avocado, and tomato. Squeeze a lime wedge over the top before serving.

Variation: If you don't have a slow cooker, soak the beans overnight, discard the soaking water, and cook everything in a heavy pot on the stove. The beans should be soft in under 2 hours, but don't wander off; you may need to add more broth every once in a while, if the soup begins to dry out.

The Immersion Blender Is My Best Friend: If you don't have the time or energy to transfer the soup contents into a blender, you can always use a handy immersion blender. Just plunk it into the pot, and it will purée a soup (or pudding, or whatever) into a dreamy, delicious dish without all the back and forth between stove and blender. It's cheap and insanely useful.

COCONUT CURRY NOODLE SOUP

g-f

veg

Curry contains turmeric, a superfood. Good for your bones, heart, liver, and immune system, turmeric is anti-inflammatory and is even known to help prevent certain cancers. Plus, it's antibacterial. Need I say more? Curry shows up in Asian, African, and Caribbean cuisine, and I think it's time we Americans started eating more of it. Go, curry!

Serves 4

1	tablespoon coconut oil
6	baby bella (or crimini) mushrooms, sliced
	Sea salt to taste
2	garlic cloves, grated
2-inch	piece of fresh ginger, grated
2	tablespoons red curry paste
2 1/2	cups vegetable stock
1	13.5-ounce can of coconut milk
3	ounces dry rice noodles (prepared according to package directions)
	Red chili pepper flakes for garnish (optional)
	Handful of fresh chopped cilantro for garnish
4	lime wedges for garnish

1. In a 2-quart pot, heat the coconut oil over medium-high heat until melted. Add the mushrooms, and season with salt. Sauté until lightly golden, 2 to 3 minutes. Add the garlic and ginger and cook until fragrant and barely golden.

2. Stir in the curry paste. Slowly pour in the vegetable stock and coconut milk, stirring constantly. Reduce the heat to low, and cook for 10 minutes.

3. To serve, divide the rice noodles among 4 deep serving bowls. Ladle the broth and mushrooms over the noodles. Top with the chili pepper, if you're using it, some cilantro, and a squeeze of fresh lime juice.

FISH CHOWDER

g-f

clean

When I was following the Body Ecology diet strictly, I made this soup all the time. This is Donna Gates's exact recipe. I. LOVE. THIS. SOUP.

Serves 2

1	tablespoon organic, unrefined coconut oil
1/2	cup leek or onion, minced
1	clove garlic, minced
1/2	cup carrots, thinly sliced
1/2	cup celery, thinly sliced
2	cups vegetable broth
1/4	cup parsley, chopped
1/2	bay leaf
1	whole clove
	A few yellow celery tops, chopped
3/4	cup white fish (sole, seabass, etc.), cut into cubes
1/8	teaspoon kelp powder
1/8	teaspoon sea salt, or to taste
2	tablespoons parsley or chives, minced

1. Sauté leek or onion and garlic in oil over low heat. Add carrots and celery and continue to sauté for several minutes. Add broth, cover, and simmer until vegetables are partially tender, about 5 minutes. Add parsley, bay leaf, clove, celery tops, and fish. Simmer 3 minutes more. Add kelp and sea salt and remove bay leaf. Serve with minced parsley or chives.

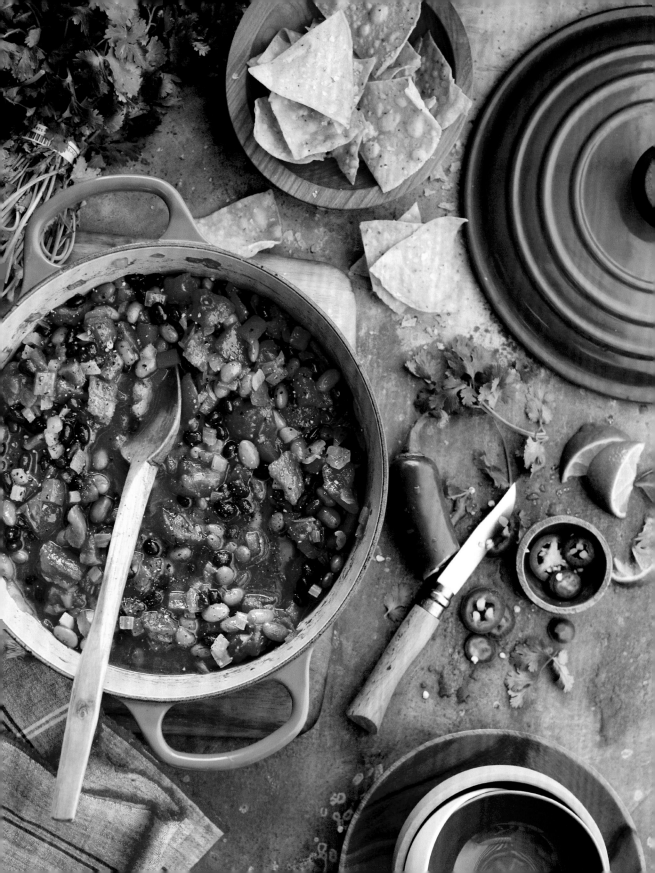

HEARTY BEAN CHILI

g-f

veg

clean

I love this recipe because it's simple, delicious, and flexible. If I have friends coming over, I can always add a little meat to satisfy their cravings. Also, this chili freezes really well. I make a big batch in the summer, freeze some, and then thaw it out on an autumn night when I don't feel like cooking.

Serves 4

- 2 tablespoons extra-virgin olive oil
- 1 medium onion, chopped
- 2 garlic cloves, chopped
- 1 red bell pepper, chopped
- 2 celery stalks, chopped fine
- 1 teaspoon sea salt
- 2 14.5-ounce cans diced tomatoes
- 1 15-ounce can black beans, drained and rinsed
- 1 15-ounce can pinto beans, drained and rinsed
- 2 teaspoons ground cumin
  Handful of fresh cilantro, chopped (plus more to garnish)
- 1 jalapeño pepper, chopped fine
- 1/4 teaspoon cayenne

1. In a 4-quart deep pot, heat the oil over medium heat. Add the onion, garlic, bell pepper, and celery. Season with salt. Sauté until the onion and garlic become lightly golden, and all of the vegetables slightly tender, 1 to 2 minutes.

2. Stir in the tomatoes, beans, cumin, cilantro, jalapeño, and cayenne. Bring to a boil. Reduce heat to medium-low, keeping the chili at a vigorous simmer (little bubbles will pop to the surface). Cook for 15 minutes more. Ladle the chili into deep serving bowls and garnish with cilantro, if desired, before serving.

WATERMELON SOUP

g-f

veg

This soup is the perfect dish on a hot summer day. It's quick and easy and will put a huge smile on your face.

Serves 4 to 6

4	cups watermelon in large cubes and $^1/_3$ cup diced (for garnish)
1	cup strawberries, topped and sliced in half
$^1/_3$	cup apple juice concentrate (thawed)
1	tablespoon fresh mint leaves
$^1/_8$	teaspoon cayenne (or less, if you don't like the heat)
	Mint sprigs for garnish

I. In a blender or food processor, process cubed watermelon, strawberries, apple juice concentrate, mint leaves, and cayenne until smooth. Refrigerate, covered, for one hour to let the flavors blend. Serve in small, chilled bowls and garnish with diced watermelon and a sprig of mint.

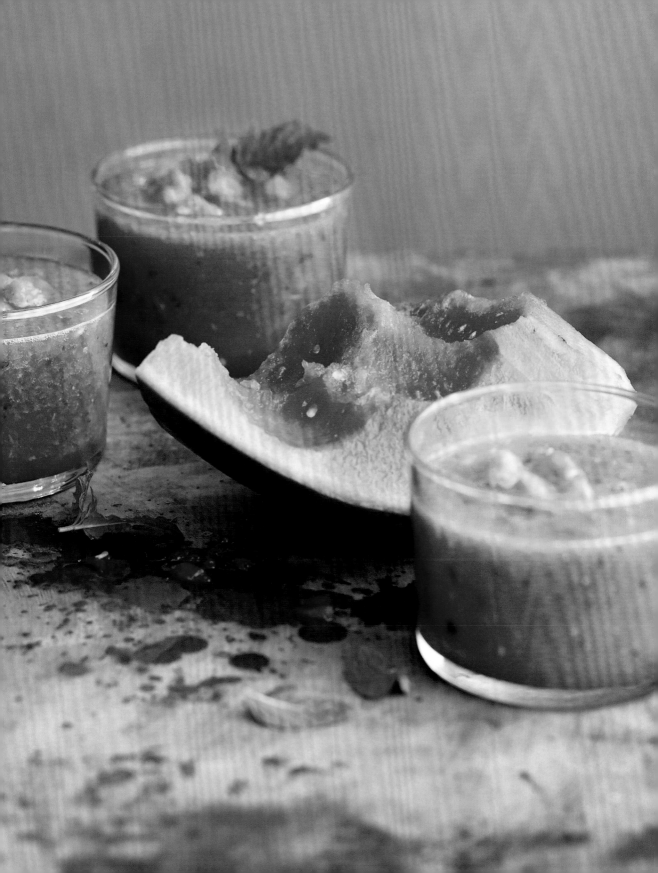

ASPARAGUS SOUP

g-f

clean

This is also from *The Body Ecology Diet.* It is creamy, elegant, and soooo good for you.

Serves 4

1 to 2	tablespoons organic, unrefined coconut oil
3 to 4	large yellow onions, chopped
5	cups chicken broth
1 1/2	pounds fresh asparagus, with tops cut off and set aside, stalks cut into 1-inch pieces (cut and discard tough ends)
	Sea salt to taste
	Pepper to taste

I. Sauté onions in oil until soft and golden. Heat broth and add cooked onions and asparagus stalk pieces. Cook on low heat until asparagus is soft. While cooking, add sea salt and pepper. Purée, then return to heat and add asparagus tops. Cook for 10 more minutes (take off heat before tops become too soft). For a cool soup, refrigerate.

CREAMY DILLED
CAULIFLOWER SOUP

g-f

veg

clean

Cauliflower gets no respect, which is too bad because it's versatile and nutritious and has tons of flavor. This is another of my favorite recipes from *The Body Ecology Diet*.

Serves 6 to 8

1	tablespoon organic, unrefined coconut oil
1	large onion, chopped
4 to 6	cloves garlic, or to taste, chopped
1	large head (or two small heads) cauliflower, cut into chunks (reserve a handful of florets)
6	tablespoons fresh dill or 2 tablespoons dried
4 to 6	cups water
	Sea salt or Herbamare to taste

1. In a stockpot, warm oil and dill, if you are using dried drill. Add onion, sautéing until translucent. Add garlic and sauté for a few minutes, being careful not to overcook it. Add cauliflower chunks (and dill if you are using fresh dill) and enough water to cover. Simmer until tender. Purée in blender and then return to stockpot. Add approximately 4 cups water depending on desired thickness of soup (thicker and creamier is usually preferred). Add sea salt or Herbamare to taste, and florets. Simmer until florets are tender. Adjust seasonings and serve.

Variation: After blending, add a handful of fresh shiitake mushroom slices and cook about 10 minutes more.

Main Dishes

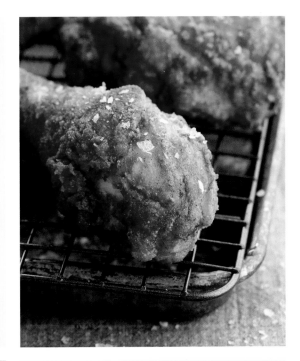

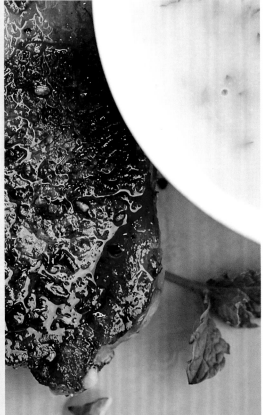

I call this section "Main Dishes" because that's how we're accustomed to describing our meals, but remember that high-quality protein is no longer the main attraction; vegetables and other whole foods should be stealing the limelight! With that said, this section gives you the chance to play with beef, beans, seafood, poultry, and more. These recipes are absolutely delicious.

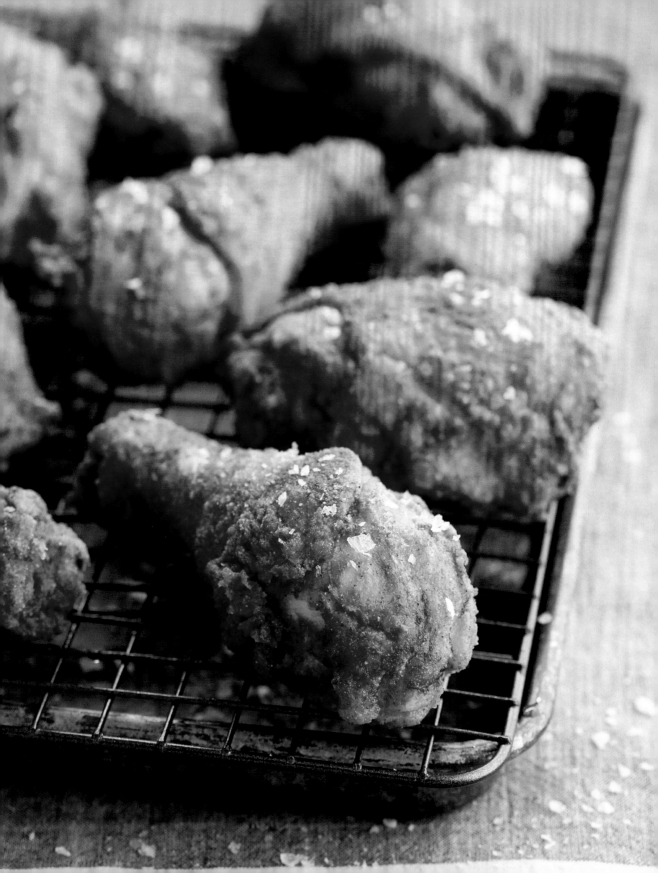

"BUTTERMILK" FRIED CHICKEN

 fun   I love fried chicken; it's a comfort food that makes me and all my guests happy. And this recipe is about as healthy as it gets. Enjoy!

Makes 10 pieces

FOR THE "BUTTERMILK" BRINE:

- 1 3/4 cups unsweetened cashew milk (it's the best of the non-dairy milks for this recipe)
- 2 tablespoons apple cider vinegar
- 1 teaspoon paprika
- 1 teaspoon sea salt

    Freshly ground black pepper to taste
- 1 3-pound whole chicken, cut up (ask your butcher to cut the breasts in half, too)

FOR THE COATING:

- 1 cup spelt or whole wheat flour
- 1 teaspoon sea salt, plus more for finishing
- 1 teaspoon paprika
- 1/2 teaspoon garlic powder

    Safflower oil for frying

---

1. Make the brine: Add the cashew milk and apple cider vinegar to a resealable plastic bag; let the bag sit open for five minutes to sour the milk. Add the paprika, salt, pepper, and chicken. Seal the bag closed and store in the refrigerator for at least 4 hours, or overnight.

---

2. Line a rimmed baking sheet with paper towels. Remove the chicken from the brine and place the pieces in a single layer on the tray. Use additional paper towels to pat the chicken dry.

---

3. Make the coating: Add the flour, salt, paprika, and garlic powder to a pie plate or deep dish. Stir until well blended. Press the chicken, one piece at a time, into the flour mixture; turn to coat the other side. Place the coated chicken pieces on a dish in a single layer, and let stand for 15 minutes. Don't skip this step. Letting the chicken sit allows the flour coating to adhere well.

---

4. Place a cooling rack inside a rimmed baking sheet; set aside.

---

continued on next page

5. Meanwhile, heat 1 inch of safflower oil in a deep skillet until the oil is simmering. Add the chicken, making sure not to crowd the pan (you'll need to fry in batches). Cook each piece without disturbing it until it is a deep golden brown underneath, about 15 minutes. Turn and cook on the other side until it is a deep golden brown and registers 165°F with an instant-read thermometer, 10 to 15 minutes more. Remove from the skillet and place on the cooling rack (this ensures a crispy bottom). Sprinkle with salt, if desired. Serve hot.

LAMB BURGERS *with*
MINT AIOLI

g-f

clean

Mm . . . the only way to improve a lamb burger is to serve it with minty-tasting aioli. It makes for an elegant combination of flavors.

FOR THE AIOLI:

1	large egg yolk
2	tablespoons freshly squeezed lemon juice (about 2 lemons)
1/4	teaspoon sea salt
1/2	teaspoon Dijon mustard
1	garlic clove
3/4	cup extra-virgin olive oil
	Handful of fresh mint, chopped

FOR THE BURGERS:

1	pound ground lamb
	Sea salt and freshly ground black pepper
	Extra-virgin olive oil
4	romaine lettuce leaves
4	tomato slices

1. To make the aioli, add the following in this exact order to the cup of an immersion blender: the egg yolk, 1 tablespoon of lemon juice, salt, mustard, garlic, and oil. Let the ingredients sit for 1 minute, until the egg yolk settles to the bottom. Place the immersion blender into the cup and slowly start pulsing the mixture. In a few seconds you will see the aioli begin to form at the bottom and little white bubbles float to the top. Move the immersion blender up and down slowly to finish. The whole process should take about 1 minute. Stir the remaining tablespoon of lemon juice and the mint into the aioli. This can be prepared up to 3 days in advance—store in an airtight container in the fridge until ready to use.

2. To make the burgers, divide the lamb into four equal portions. Shape into patties, and season with salt and pepper. In a 12-inch cast iron skillet, heat 1 teaspoon of oil over medium-high

continued on next page

heat until shimmering. Add the patties to the skillet. Cook until the meat achieves desired doneness, turning halfway through cooking (8 to 10 minutes for medium-rare).

3. To serve, place one burger in the middle of a romaine leaf. Top with a tomato slice. Drizzle aioli on top. Serve hot.

CATFISH TACOS *with*
SPICY RED CABBAGE SLAW

*g-f**

I love a good taco, and this recipe combines delicious, fresh fish with crispy vegetables and bright, vibrant flavors. If you like, you can also serve these tacos with the Tofu Sour Cream on page 163.

Serves 4

8	corn or flour tortillas
1/4	cup plus 2 teaspoons extra-virgin olive oil
2	tablespoons freshly squeezed lime juice (about 2 limes)
	Sea salt
1/2	of a small head of red cabbage, thinly shredded
1	serrano pepper, minced
	Handful of fresh cilantro, chopped
14	ounces catfish fillet (preferably one whole fillet)
	Freshly ground black pepper
	Toppings, as desired (avocado, salsa, lime wedges, fresh cilantro)

1. Preheat the oven to 250°F. Stack the tortillas in the center of a sheet of foil. Wrap loosely to close. Place in the oven to heat while you prepare the fish and slaw. Alternatively, you can heat the tortillas on a grill just before you're ready to serve the tacos.

2. Prepare the slaw: In a medium bowl, whisk 1/4 cup of the olive oil and the lime juice until well combined. Season with salt. Add the cabbage, serrano pepper, and cilantro; toss until fully coated. Let sit at room temperature while you cook the fish.

3. Season the fillet with salt and pepper.

4. In a 10-inch nonstick skillet, heat 2 teaspoons of oil over medium-high heat until shimmer-

continued on next page

* GLUTEN-FREE IF YOU USE CORN TORTILLAS.

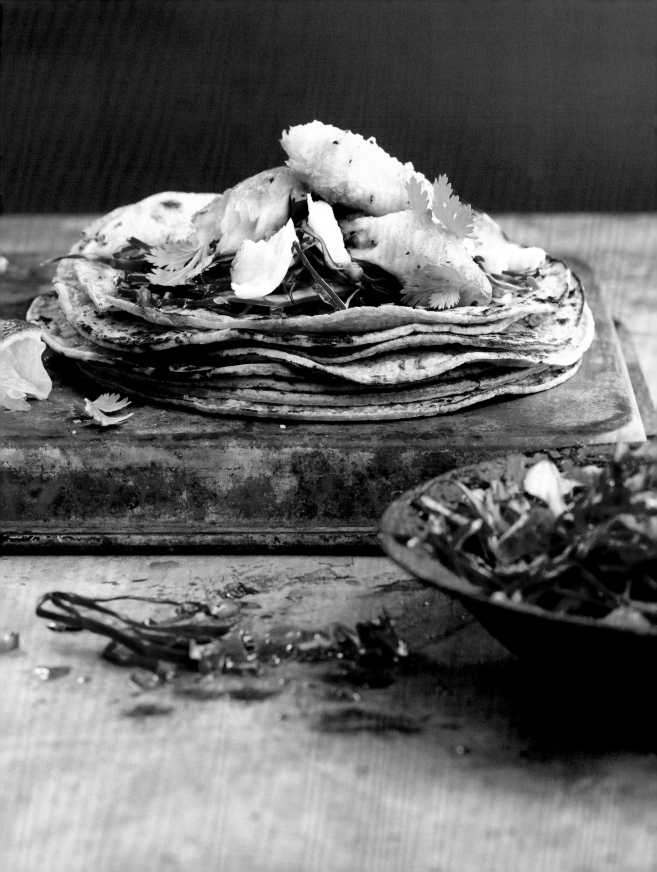

ing. Carefully place the fish in the pan. Cook, undisturbed, until lightly golden on the underside, 6 to 7 minutes. Turn the fish over and continue cooking until lightly golden and opaque in the center, 6 to 7 minutes more depending on thickness.

5.   To serve, arrange the catfish, slaw, and desired toppings on a large platter. Serve family style, letting everyone assemble their own tacos.

LAMB LOLLIPOPS &
MINTY YOGURT SAUCE

I love the look, and the delicacy, of lamb lollipops. This dish also has a minty condiment, but this time it's got the gentle kick of fresh jalapeño. It gives this whole dish another dimension.

Serves 4

8	3/4-inch-thick lamb chops, frenched
	Sea salt and freshly ground black pepper
	A few sprigs of fresh thyme (stems discarded and leaves chopped)
	Extra-virgin olive oil
6	ounces plain coconut milk yogurt
	Freshly grated zest and squeezed juice of 1 lime
12	fresh mint leaves, chopped
1/2	jalapeño pepper, seeded and minced
	Splash of soy sauce or tamari

1. Season both sides of the lamb chops with the salt, pepper, and thyme. Heat a 10-inch cast iron skillet over medium-high heat. Drizzle in enough oil to coat the bottom of the pan. Add the lamb chops, and cook, undisturbed, until deep golden brown underneath, 3 to 4 minutes. Turn and cook until browned on the other side, 2 to 3 minutes more. Remove the pan from the heat, and let the lamb chops sit for 1 minute.

2. In a small bowl, combine the yogurt, lime zest and juice, mint, jalapeño, and soy sauce (or tamari). Whisk until well blended. Season with salt.

3. Arrange 2 lamb chops on each dish. Spoon sauce on top, and serve immediately.

What are frenched lamb chops? "Frenching" is a butchering technique that removes the meat, fat, and membranes connecting the individual ribs. This gives the ribs a clean and elegant look. You can find frenched ribs at the butcher, better grocers, and most Whole Foods Markets.

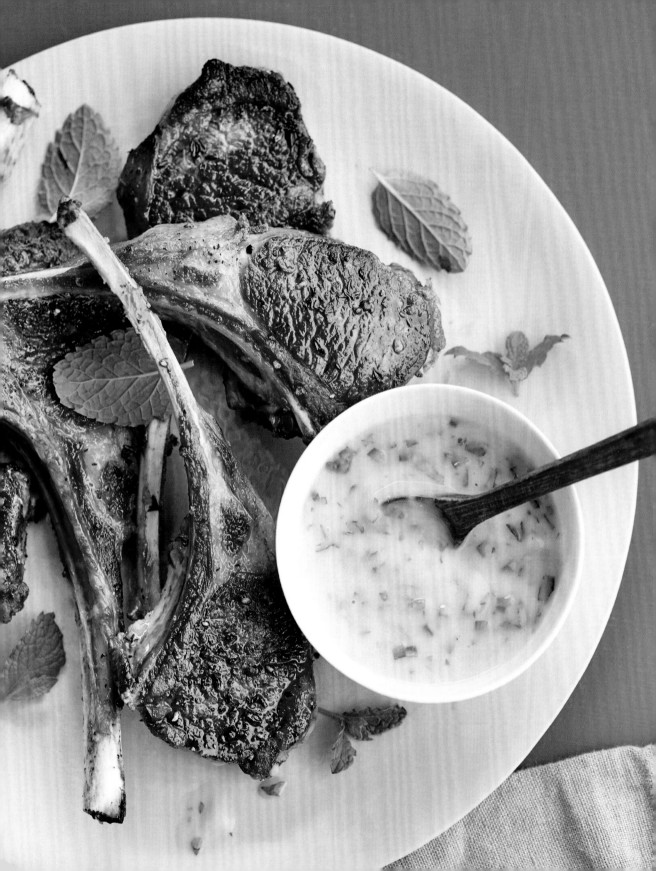

LENTIL "MEATLOAF" & SHIITAKE MUSHROOM GRAVY

Beans are so good for you, but many of us don't know how to make them scrumptiously delicious. Until now . . .

Serves 4

FOR THE "MEATLOAF":

1	15-ounce can lentils, drained
	Handful of fresh flat-leaf parsley, chopped
3	garlic cloves
1/2	teaspoon sea salt
	Freshly ground black pepper to taste
1	tablespoon soy sauce or tamari
2	teaspoons Dijon mustard
1	large egg
1/2	cup panko breadcrumbs (preferably whole wheat)

FOR THE GRAVY:

2	teaspoons extra-virgin olive oil
7	ounces shiitake mushrooms, caps thinly sliced (stems removed and discarded)
1	small onion, grated
2	teaspoons whole wheat pastry flour
1	cup vegetable stock
	Splash of soy sauce or tamari
	Sea salt and freshly ground black pepper to taste

1. Preheat the oven to 375°F. Line an 8 x 4 x 2-inch loaf pan with a sheet of parchment paper long enough to hang over the sides of the pan.

* FOR A GLUTEN-FREE VERSION, USE GLUTEN-FREE BREADCRUMBS AND SUBSTITUTE 1 TEASPOON OF CORNSTARCH FOR THE 2 TEASPOONS OF WHOLE WHEAT PASTRY FLOUR. ALSO, USE TAMARI INSTEAD OF SOY SAUCE.

2.　In the bowl of a food processor, combine the lentils, parsley, garlic, salt, pepper, soy sauce (or tamari), mustard, egg, and breadcrumbs. Pulse until the ingredients are well mixed and the lentils are mostly puréed (it's okay to have a few whole pieces). Spread the mixture into the prepared loaf pan.

3.　Bake for 30 minutes. Let the loaf cool for 5 to 10 minutes before slicing it into 8 pieces.

4.　Meanwhile, prepare the gravy. In an 8-inch skillet, heat the oil over medium-high heat until shimmering. Add the mushrooms and onion. Sauté until lightly golden, 3 to 4 minutes. Sprinkle the flour over the mixture. Stir until the mushrooms and onion are well coated, adding one more teaspoon of oil if the pan seems too dry. Slowly add the vegetable stock while stirring. The gravy will begin to thicken quickly. Reduce the heat to low and let cook, stirring constantly, for 2 minutes. Add the soy sauce (or tamari), and season with the salt and pepper.

5.　To serve, arrange 2 pieces of the lentil loaf on each plate, spooning gravy over the top. Serve immediately.

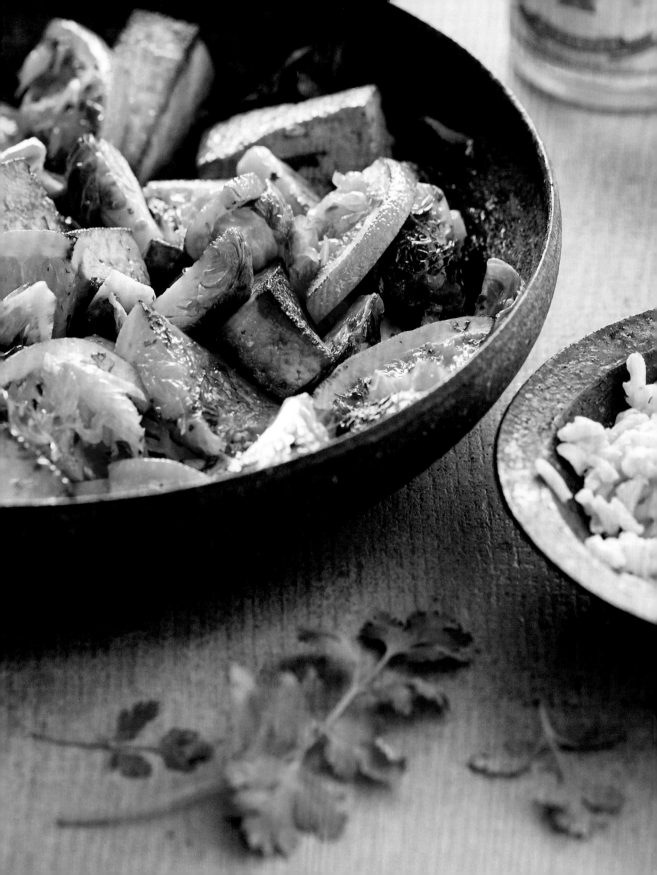

ORANGE & SESAME STIR-FRIED TOFU
with BRUSSELS SPROUTS

g-f*

veg

clean

I like tofu best when it's marinated, picking up lots of flavor, and then fried, so it's got a slightly crispy texture. Throw in some veggies and serve over brown rice, and you've got a great meal that even your carnivorous friends will love.

Serves 4

2	oranges, cut into 1/4-inch-thick triangles
3	garlic cloves, smashed
1/3	cup soy sauce or tamari
2	tablespoons sesame oil
	Sea salt and freshly ground black pepper to taste
1	pound extra-firm organic tofu, drained and cubed (see Tia Tip)
	Handful of fresh cilantro, chopped
3	tablespoons extra-virgin olive oil
12	ounces Brussels sprouts, cut into quarters

1. In a deep bowl, mash the oranges to release some of the juices (a bar muddler works perfectly for this). Add the garlic, soy sauce (or tamari), sesame oil, salt, and pepper. Stir with a fork to combine. Add the tofu and cilantro and toss well with a rubber spatula to coat. Let sit, covered, in the refrigerator for 2 hours, or overnight.

2. Use a slotted spoon to remove the tofu and orange slices, reserving the marinating liquid.

3. In a wok or deep skillet, heat 2 tablespoons of the olive oil. Add the tofu. Cook over high heat until nicely browned on all sides, adding the remaining tablespoon of olive oil, if needed, to keep the tofu from sticking to the pan. Transfer to a dish to keep warm (you may need to do this in two batches depending on the size of your wok or skillet). Add the Brussels sprouts to the skillet. Sauté until golden and tender, about 5 minutes, adding more olive oil 1 teaspoon at a time if the

continued on next page

* GLUTEN-FREE IF YOU USE TAMARI.

WHOLE NEW YOU

pan seems too dry. Stir in the orange slices. Return the tofu to the wok, along with the reserved marinating liquid. Stir until everything is well mixed. Sauté 2 more minutes. Serve hot.

Tia Tip: Draining tofu: Tofu sold in stores is preserved in water, so it absorbs a lot of it. If you want tofu to really absorb the seasonings and flavors of the dish you're making, it's important to get rid of some of this excess water. Here's how: Remove the tofu from the package. Wrap it loosely in 1 or 2 paper towels and place it on a baking sheet (with rims). Place a cutting board on top of the tofu and a couple of weights on top of the cutting board; books or heavy plates are good. Let the tofu "press" for 15 to 30 minutes. You will see liquid absorbing into the paper towels and even running off onto the baking sheet. This pressed tofu will hold lots of flavor!

MOROCCAN CHICKEN *with*
LEMON & OLIVES

Chicken doesn't need a whole lot of fancy treatment to be delicious. This recipe is simple, elegant, and tastes great.

Serves 4 to 6

3¹/2	pound chicken, cut into pieces (your butcher can do this for you)
	Extra-virgin olive oil
	Sea salt to taste
1	large yellow onion, sliced
20	pitted green olives
2	lemons, cut into 1/4-inch-thick slices
2	teaspoons cumin
1	teaspoon coriander

1. Preheat the oven to 425°F.

2. Arrange the chicken in a 9 x 13-inch deep roasting pan. Drizzle a bit of oil all over. Season generously with salt. Roast for 25 minutes.

3. Meanwhile, add the onion, olives, lemons, cumin, and coriander to a medium bowl. Drizzle in a few teaspoons of oil, and toss to mix well. Scatter the mixture over the chicken in the roasting pan. Roast 25 to 30 minutes more, basting with the pan juices occasionally, until the chicken thighs register 165°F. Serve hot.

PAN-ROASTED CHICKEN *with* MAPLE BACON SAUCE

 g-f ✳ This recipe is great for entertaining and can be served family style by bringing the pan to the table. It looks beautiful, making it worth the extra work of browning the chicken and buying a specialty ingredient like sherry vinegar.

Serves 4

8	chicken thighs
2	teaspoons sea salt, plus more to taste
4	slices bacon, chopped
1	medium onion, sliced
1	tablespoon soy sauce or tamari
1	tablespoon pure maple syrup
1	teaspoon Dijon mustard
1	tablespoon sherry vinegar
	Handful of fresh flat-leaf parsley, chopped

1. Season the chicken with 2 teaspoons of salt; set aside.

2. Heat a 10-inch deep skillet over medium-high heat. Add the bacon, and cook until crispy. Transfer the cooked bacon to a paper towel–lined plate to drain. Spoon the oil from the pan into a heatproof container.

3. Add 1 tablespoon of oil back to the pan over medium-high heat. Add 4 pieces of chicken to the pan, skin side down. Cook, undisturbed, until the underside is a deep golden color, 5 to 7 minutes. Turn the chicken and cook on the other side until deep golden, about 5 minutes more. Transfer to a dish. Repeat with the remaining pieces of uncooked chicken, adding more of the reserved oil, if needed, to prevent it from sticking to the pan. Set the browned chicken aside while you prepare the sauce. (Note: The chicken is not cooked through yet; it'll finish cooking in the sauce.)

continued on next page

✳ GLUTEN-FREE IF YOU USE TAMARI.

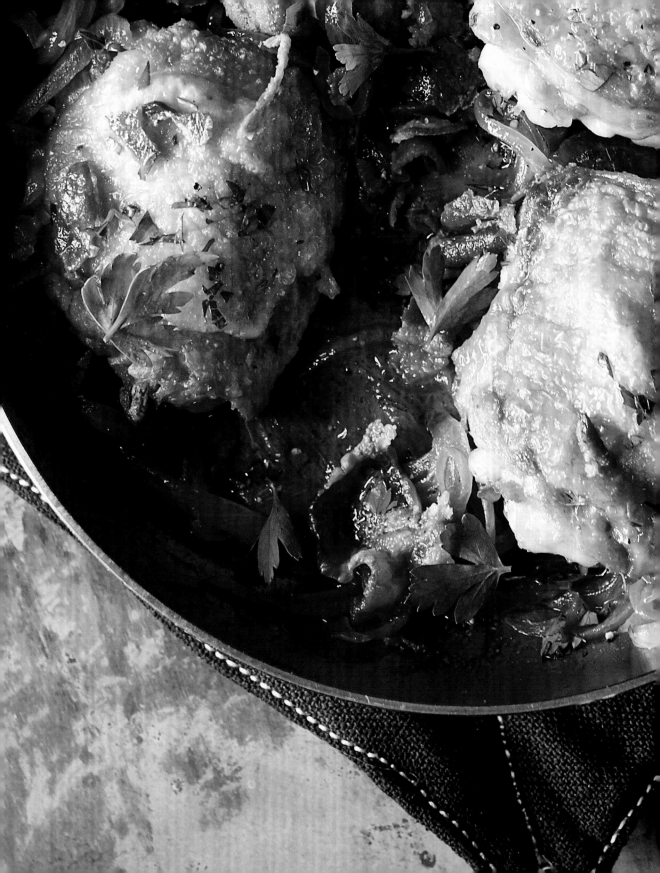

4. Add the onion slices to the skillet over medium heat. Season with salt. Sauté until golden and tender, 3 to 4 minutes, stirring occasionally so they don't stick to the pan.

5. Meanwhile, add the soy sauce (or tamari), syrup, mustard, and vinegar to a small bowl; whisk to combine. Stir the mixture along with a 1/2 cup of water into the skillet with the onions. Bring to a boil. Add the chicken back to the pan and spoon the juices over the top. Reduce the heat to a simmer. Cook, uncovered, for 20 to 25 minutes, until the chicken is cooked through.

6. Sprinkle the cooked bacon pieces and parsley on top. Serve hot.

Variation: If you'd like to skip the bacon, sprinkle 1 to 2 tablespoons of olive oil on the chicken instead.

Tia Tip: I don't recommend making this dish in advance, since the chicken skin will get rubbery when reheated.

ROASTED COD *with*
OLIVES, TOMATOES, & GARLIC

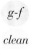

g-f

clean

Cod is a delicate fish and shouldn't be overwhelmed by other seasonings. This dish brings together classic Mediterranean flavors that support and enhance cod's natural taste. Delish.

Serves 4

1 1/2	pounds cod fillet
	Sea salt and freshly ground black pepper
1	pint grape tomatoes, cut in half
2	ounces pitted kalamata olives, cut in half
3	garlic cloves, chopped
2 to 3	tablespoons extra-virgin olive oil
	Handful of fresh flat-leaf parsley, chopped

1. Preheat the oven to 375°F. Line an 11 x 17-inch rimmed baking pan with a sheet of parchment paper long enough to hang over the sides.

2. Arrange the fillets in a single layer on the prepared pan. Season with salt and pepper. Scatter the tomatoes, olives, and garlic over the fish. Drizzle the olive oil on top. Bake for 30 to 35 minutes, spooning the juices over the fish halfway through until it is opaque and flakes easily with the tip of a fork.

3. Transfer the fish to a large serving platter. Scatter the chopped parsley on top. Serve immediately, family style.

ROASTED CORNISH HENS &
RED POTATOES

I learned this dish as a kid because my mother made it all the time. It's almost a whole meal: a delicious bird, surrounded by its own side dish. Just add a salad, and you have a gourmet-ish meal that is really *easy*. It's perfect for a mom on the go, and the whole family will love it. By the way, this recipe assumes that each hen will feed two people—Cornish heans are a lot bigger today than they were when I was a kid! If you find Cornish hens that don't seem big enough to serve two, adjust the recipe accordingly.

Serves 4

2	whole Cornish hens (or 4, depending on size)
1 to 2	tablespoons extra-virgin olive oil (plus more to drizzle)
	Sea salt and freshly ground black pepper
3 to 4	red potatoes, cut into wedges
4-inch	piece of fresh rosemary

1. Preheat the oven to 425°F.

2. Place the hens on an 11 x 17-inch rimmed baking sheet. Drizzle a bit of oil over them and season with salt and pepper all over.

3. In a medium bowl, toss the potatoes with 1 to 2 tablespoons of oil. Season with salt and pepper. Hold the rosemary sprig at the top with one hand, and use your pointer finger and thumb to strip the needles off the branch. Add the needles to the potatoes, and give it all a good toss. Spread the potatoes in a single layer onto the baking sheet with the hens.

4. Roast for 1 hour, turning the potatoes halfway through, until the hens register 165°F and the potatoes are golden and crisp all around. Serve hot.

SHRIMP COBB SALAD

 g-f

A Cobb salad makes me feel like I'm having a ladies' lunch in a fancy hotel. This recipe is served family style, so everyone can take their favorite ingredients. But I like them all!

Serves 4

FOR THE SALAD:

12	ounces large shrimp, peeled and deveined
1	head Boston lettuce, chopped
1	heart romaine lettuce, chopped
1	pint grape tomatoes, cut in half
4	hard-boiled eggs, cut in half
8	slices cooked bacon, crumbled
1	avocado, pitted and chopped

FOR THE DRESSING:

1/4	cup red wine vinegar
	Sea salt and freshly ground black pepper to taste
2	teaspoons whole grain mustard
1	teaspoon honey
1/2	cup extra-virgin olive oil

1. Fill a 2-quart pot with water and bring to a boil over high heat. Add the shrimp, remove the pot from heat, cover it tightly with a lid, and set aside for 10 minutes. Drain the shrimp and plunge them into a bowl with ice water to stop the cooking process; set aside. FYI: You can cook the shrimp up to 2 days before making the salad, as long as they are refrigerated.

2. Arrange the lettuces, tomatoes, eggs, bacon, avocado, and shrimp in rows on a large platter to serve the salad family style.

3. Prepare the dressing: Add the vinegar, salt, pepper, mustard, honey, and oil to a deep bowl. Whisk vigorously to combine. Spoon the dressing over the top of the salad, or serve it in a bowl on the side. Refrigerate any excess dressing in a sealed container; it will last for a week.

continued on next page

Tia Tip: How to boil an egg: If you're new to the kitchen, here's a tried-and-true method for making a hard-boiled egg: Place 4 eggs in a small pot with enough water to cover them. Bring it to a boil over high heat. Remove from heat, cover with a lid, and let sit for 10 minutes. Drain the water and set the eggs in a bowl of cold water to stop the cooking process. Hard-boiled eggs can stay in the fridge for up to a week, and I find they're easier to peel after a day or two.

SALMON CROQUETTES

g-f *

These croquettes are lovely and elegant. Easy to make, they're great to serve for lunch or as an appetizer at a dinner party.

Serves 4

2	6-ounce cans wild pink salmon
1	small onion, chopped fine
1	tablespoon Dijon mustard
1	celery stalk, chopped fine
1/4	teaspoon paprika
	Handful of fresh flat-leaf parsley, chopped
1	large egg
	Sea salt and freshly ground black pepper to taste
1	cup whole wheat breadcrumbs (or gluten-free)
	Coconut oil for frying

1. Add the salmon, onion, mustard, celery, paprika, parsley, egg, salt, pepper, and 1/2 cup of the breadcrumbs to a food processor. Pulse until the mixture is blended but still has some chunks of salmon. Cover and chill in the fridge for at least 1 hour, or overnight.

2. When you are ready to cook the croquettes, divide the mixture into 8 even balls. You can flatten then into patties or form them into little sticks. Use the remaining 1/2 cup of breadcrumbs to coat the croquettes all around.

3. In a 10-inch skillet, melt a few tablespoons of coconut oil over medium heat. Once the oil is shimmering and fragrant, add the croquettes to the pan (you may need to do this in batches, so as not to overcrowd the pan). Cook until golden underneath, 3 to 4 minutes. Turn the croquettes and cook until golden on the other side, 3 to 4 minutes more. Serve hot.

* GLUTEN-FREE IF YOU USE GLUTEN-FREE BREADCRUMBS.

SHRIMP & BROCCOLI
GINGER STIR-FRY

g-f*

I love shrimp. And broccoli. So putting them together, with lovely flavors, makes me happy. Served over quinoa, this dish makes for a really balanced, satisfying meal.

Serves 4

1/4	cup chicken stock
1/4	cup soy sauce or tamari
1	tablespoon sesame oil
1	teaspoon agave syrup (or more, to taste)
	Freshly ground black pepper
1	tablespoon extra-virgin olive oil (plus more as needed)
2	garlic cloves, chopped
1-inch	piece of fresh ginger, peeled and chopped fine
1	pound large shrimp, peeled and deveined
1	head of broccoli (florets only, save stalks for another use)
2	teaspoons cornstarch
2	cups cooked quinoa

1. Add the stock, soy sauce (or tamari), sesame oil, agave syrup, and pepper to a small bowl. Whisk to combine; set aside.

2. Heat the oil in a wok or 12-inch skillet until shimmering. Add the garlic and ginger. Sauté until lightly golden, about 1 minute. Add the shrimp to the pan. Sauté until just cooked through (be careful not to overcook the shrimp to avoid toughness), about 5 minutes. Transfer the shrimp to a bowl.

3. Add the broccoli to the pan. Add more oil, 1 teaspoon at a time, if the pan seems too dry. Sauté until the broccoli is bright green and tender when pierced with a fork, 8 to 10 minutes.

* GLUTEN-FREE IF YOU USE TAMARI.

MAIN DISHES

4.   Reserve 1 tablespoon of the soy sauce mixture. Pour the rest into the skillet and add the shrimp. Stir until well mixed.

5.   Add the cornstarch to the reserved soy sauce mixture. Whisk until well blended and there are no visible signs of cornstarch. Stirring constantly, pour the mixture into the skillet. Cook for 1 to 2 more minutes, until the sauce has thickened a bit.

6.   Divide the quinoa among four serving bowls. Top with the shrimp, broccoli, and sauce. Serve hot.

THAI BEEF LETTUCE CUPS

g-f * This is like a lettuce taco, Thai-style. I love the juicy, rich taste of the beef, balanced by the cool crispness of the lettuce.

Serves 4

2	teaspoons extra-virgin olive oil
1	small onion, chopped fine
1	garlic clove, chopped fine
1	pound ground beef (lean 90 percent)
	Handful of fresh cilantro, chopped
2	teaspoons fish sauce
1	tablespoon soy sauce or tamari
1	teaspoon dried chili peppers, or to taste
1/2	teaspoon coconut sugar
	Sea salt to taste
1	head Boston lettuce
	Lime wedges, for garnish
	Fresh mint, for garnish

1. In a 10-inch skillet, heat the oil over medium-high heat until shimmering. Add the onion and garlic. Sauté until lightly golden, 1 to 2 minutes. Add the beef, using a fork to break up any large chunks (you want little pieces of ground meat). Add the cilantro, fish sauce, soy sauce (or tamari), chili pepper, and sugar. Reduce heat to medium-low. Continue cooking, stirring every couple of minutes, until the beef is completely cooked through, 7 to 9 minutes.

2. Meanwhile, rinse the lettuce leaves and pat them dry. Arrange the leaves on a platter.

3. Taste the cooked beef. Adjust the seasonings, adding salt and more chili pepper, if you'd like. Spoon the beef over the lettuce leaves. Garnish with lime wedges and fresh mint. Serve immediately.

Tia Tip: How to eat a lettuce cup: Squeeze a little lime juice on the beef, fold the lettuce leaf, and eat it like a taco!

* GLUTEN-FREE IF YOU USE TAMARI AND GLUTEN-FREE FISH SAUCE.

MAIN DISHES

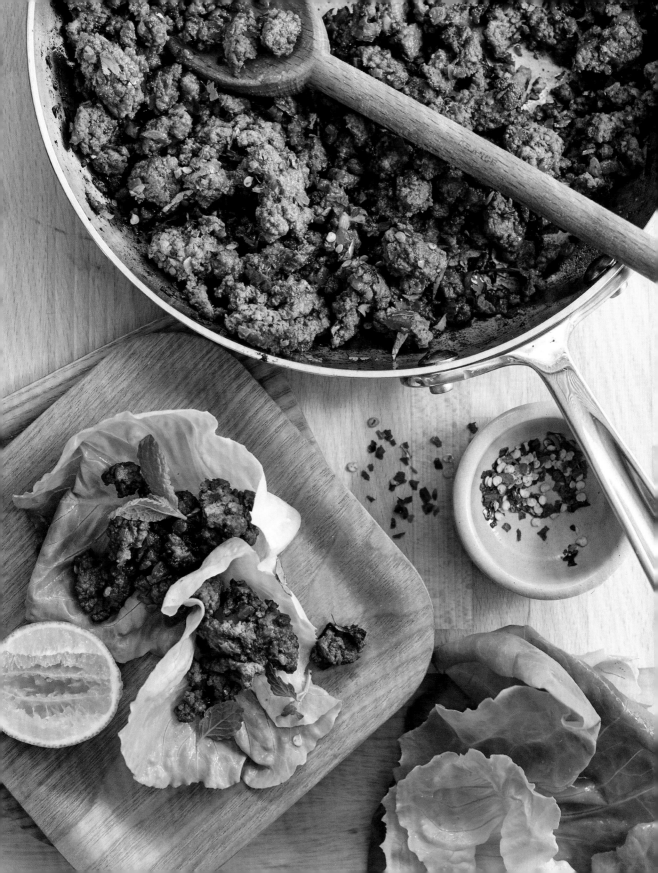

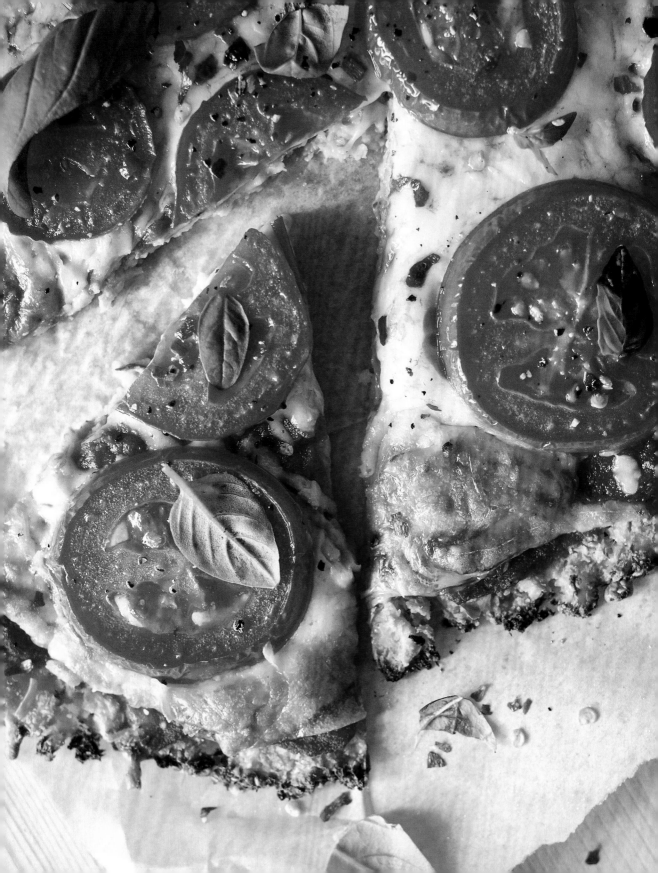

TOMATO & BASIL
CAULIFLOWER PIZZA

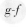

g-f

veg

I know. I know. A cauliflower crust sounds crazy, but you will be amazed by how delicious it is. If you're passing on flour but can't live without pizza, this is your answer!

Serves 2

Sea salt to taste

1   small head cauliflower

3/4   cup Daiya dairy-free, soy-free mozzarella cheese shreds

2   tablespoons Non-Dairy Parmesan "Cheese" (page 229, or Go Veggie brand)

Cooking spray

1/4   cup Roasted Marinara Sauce (page 227)

1   plum tomato, very thinly sliced

6   fresh basil leaves

1.   Fill a 4-quart pot with water. Bring to a boil over high heat. Cut the florets off the head of cauliflower (you can save the stalks for another use). Add them to the bowl of a food processor. Pulse until they look like grains of couscous. Alternately, you can do this using the smallest holes on a box grater.

2.   Salt the boiling water, and add the cauliflower grains. Cook for 2 to 3 minutes, until tender.

3.   Using a fine sieve, drain the cauliflower. Let it sit in the strainer to cool for 20 minutes.

4.   Meanwhile, adjust the oven rack to the lowest position. Place a pizza stone or steel on the rack, if you have one. Preheat the oven to 425°F.

5.   Transfer the cauliflower to a clean kitchen towel. Roll the towel up and squeeze out as much water from it as possible (you'll be surprised how much actually drains out).

6.   In a medium bowl, combine the cauliflower, 1/4 cup of mozzarella, and the Parmesan cheese. Stir with a fork until well mixed.

continued on next page

7.   Line a pizza pan with a sheet of parchment paper. Lightly grease the paper with cooking spray. Gather the cauliflower mixture into a ball and place it at the center of the parchment paper. Press it out into a 10-inch circle, making sure there are no holes in the crust. Bake for 15 minutes, until golden around the edges.

8.   Remove the pan from the oven. Spread the marinara sauce over the crust, leaving a 1/2-inch border. Sprinkle the remaining 1/2 cup of mozzarella cheese over the sauce. Top with the tomato slices. Return the pizza to the oven, and bake for 10 to 12 minutes more, until the cheese is melted and the crust is well browned. Arrange the basil on top, and serve immediately.

TURKEY MEATBALLS

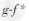

g-f* My son absolutely loves meatballs, and so do I. This is a meal that the whole family can enjoy and it's a regular favorite in our house. We serve it over zoodles or whole wheat or quinoa flour noodles.

Makes 28 meatballs

1/2	cup dairy-free milk (soy, almond, cashew, etc.)
1/2	cup old-fashioned oats (not quick cooking)
2 to 3	tablespoons extra-virgin olive oil
1	pound ground turkey
	Handful of fresh flat-leaf parsley, chopped
1	large egg, lightly beaten
1/4	cup Non-Dairy Parmesan "Cheese" (page 229)
2	garlic cloves, grated
1/4	teaspoon freshly grated nutmeg
3/4	teaspoon sea salt
	Freshly ground black pepper, as desired
	Roasted Marinara Sauce (page 227)
	Zoodles

1. Add the milk and oats to a small pot over medium heat. Cook until the milk is very hot, but not boiling. Reduce the heat to a simmer, continuing to cook until the mixture has a thick oatmeal consistency. Set aside and let the mixture cool for 5 minutes.

2. Preheat the oven to 450°F. Drizzle the oil onto a rimmed baking sheet; set aside.

3. In a large bowl combine the turkey, parsley, egg, Parmesan, garlic, nutmeg, salt, pepper, and oatmeal mixture. Using a sturdy spoon or spatula, stir until all of the ingredients are completely combined. Form the mixture into 28 equally sized meatballs. Place them onto the prepared baking sheet.

4. Bake for 25 to 30 minutes, turning at the halfway point, until the meatballs are nicely brown all around. Serve hot with marinara sauce, and zoodles, if desired.

continued on next page

* GLUTEN-FREE IF OATS ARE MARKED "GLUTEN-FREE."

Zoodles (named after zucchini noodles) are "noodles" made from vegetables, and they're easy to make. All you need is a spiral slicer—also known as a Spiralizer—an inexpensive kitchen gadget. You should be able to find one in a kitchen store or online for under fifteen dollars. Making zoodles is fun, and eating them is even better.

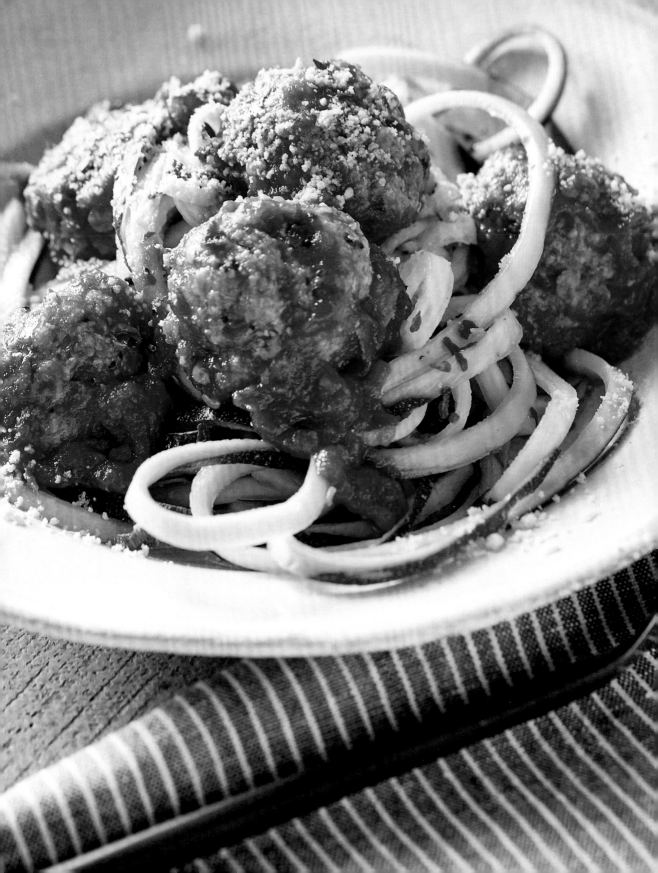

TURKEY & MUSHROOM BOLOGNESE

g-f*   I love a good Bolognese sauce. Although it's traditionally made with beef, I like to use turkey, just for fun. Between the meat, the vegetables, and the noodles, this is a hearty and satisfying dish. *Mangia!*

Serves 6 to 8

2	tablespoons extra-virgin olive oil (plus more as needed)
1	large onion, chopped fine
1	carrot, chopped fine
8	ounces mushrooms, chopped fine (white button or baby bella)
	Sea salt and freshly ground black pepper to taste
1	pound ground turkey
1	28-ounce can crushed tomatoes
1/4	teaspoon of freshly grated nutmeg
1	pound uncooked whole wheat pasta (rigatoni or fusilli)
	Non-Dairy Parmesan "Cheese," for garnish (optional, recipe on page 229)
	Handful of fresh chopped basil, for garnish

1.   In a 12-inch deep skillet, heat the oil over medium-high heat until it's shimmering. Add the onion and carrot. Cook until the onion pieces are golden, stirring occasionally, 2 to 3 minutes. Add the mushrooms and season with salt and pepper. Sauté, stirring occasionally, until the mushrooms are lightly browned, about 5 minutes. Using a slotted spoon, transfer the vegetable mixture to a plate.

2.   Add the turkey to the skillet, adding a bit more oil if the pan seems too dry. Using a mashing motion with the tines of a fork, break the turkey into tiny pieces. Cook until lightly browned. Add the vegetables back to the pan, along with the tomatoes and nutmeg. Bring the sauce to a boil. Reduce the heat to low, and let simmer for 20 minutes.

3. Meanwhile, prepare the pasta according to the package directions.

4. To serve, add the cooked pasta to the skillet. Stir until well coated with the sauce. Divide into deep serving bowls. Garnish with the cheese, if desired, and basil.

TURKEY SAUSAGE & PEPPERS

Have you noticed I love turkey? Especially turkey sausages. This is a lovely, stewy dish that will keep you warm and happy.

Serves 4

1	tablespoon extra-virgin olive oil (plus more as needed)
8	Italian-style turkey sausages (mild or spicy)
2	green bell peppers, seeded and sliced
2	red bell peppers, seeded and sliced
1	large yellow onion, thinly sliced
	Sea salt to taste
1	14-ounce can crushed tomatoes
1 1/2	cups chicken stock
1 to 2	teaspoons dried basil
1/2	teaspoon red chili pepper flakes

I. In a deep 12-inch skillet, heat the oil over medium-high heat. Add the sausages. Cook until nicely browned all around, 8 to 10 minutes. Transfer the sausages to a plate; set aside.

2. Add the peppers and onion to the skillet. Season with salt. Using a wooden spoon, scrape up any browned bits at the bottom of the pan. Reduce the heat to medium-low. Sauté the peppers and onion, stirring occasionally, until golden and tender, 15 to 20 minutes, adding more oil, 1 teaspoon at a time, if the pan seems too dry.

3. Add the tomatoes, stock, basil, and chili pepper. Stir to combine. Return the sausages to the pan, pouring in any juices that have collected on the dish. Increase the heat to medium-high and bring to a boil. Reduce heat to a simmer. Cook for 20 minutes more. Taste for seasoning, adding more salt and chili flakes if desired. Serve hot.

MAIN DISHES

* GLUTEN-FREE IF SAUSAGES ARE GLUTEN-FREE.

NOURISH BOWL

We discovered a version of this dish in New York City while Cory was promoting the movie *American Sniper*. Quinoa has become quite a popular ingredient, but I had never seen it served with an egg. I was instantly impressed by the many different textures and flavors of the combination: the quinoa is chewy and nutty, while the shiitake mushrooms are earthy and almost meaty. The egg gives it a heartiness and substance, while the collards lift the whole dish with their crispy, green crunch. I was so taken with it, I went ahead and created a kicked-up version that includes hot sauce—yum! This is a great dish to serve at any meal. Use the cinnamon when you make it for breakfast!

Serves 4

1	cup quinoa
2	cups vegetable broth
1	garlic clove, grated
1/2	teaspoon cinnamon (optional)
2	splashes of soy sauce or tamari
	Sea salt to taste
2	tablespoons extra-virgin olive oil (plus more as needed)
6	ounces shiitake mushrooms, caps thinly sliced (remove and discard the stems)
	Freshly ground black pepper
4	large eggs
	Crispy Collard Chips (page 194)
	Hot sauce to taste (optional)

1. In a medium pot, add the quinoa, broth, garlic, cinnamon (if you're using it), and soy sauce (or tamari). Season with salt. Cook over medium-high heat until the mixture begins to boil. Reduce the heat to medium-low. Cook until the liquid has been absorbed, about 15 minutes.

2. Meanwhile, in a 10-inch skillet, heat 2 tablespoons of oil over medium-high heat. Add the mushrooms. Season with salt and pepper. Cook, shaking the pan once or twice (no need to stir

continued on next page

* GLUTEN-FREE IF YOU USE TAMARI.

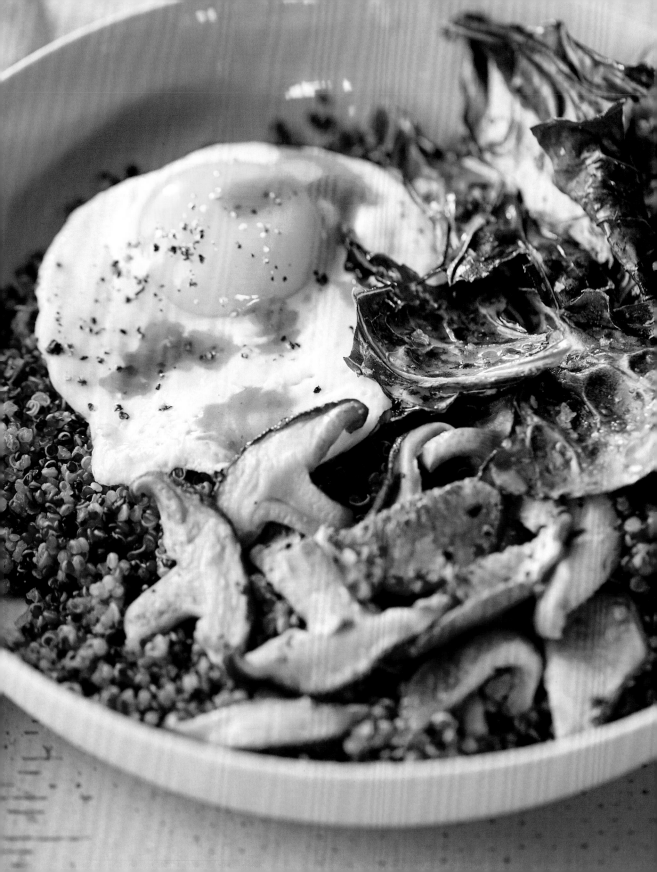

the mushrooms vigorously as they won't brown well if you fuss with them too much), until the mushrooms are tender and lightly golden, about 5 minutes. Transfer them to a dish and set aside.

3.   Return the skillet to the stove over medium-low heat. Add a few more drops of oil to the pan. Crack the eggs, one at a time, into the skillet. Cook until the edges crisp up and the egg whites look set, 3 to 4 minutes.

4.   Divide the cooked quinoa between four deep bowls. Top each bowl with shiitake mushrooms, collard chips, 1 egg, and a few dashes of hot sauce, if desired. Serve immediately.

CHICKPEA BURGERS

g-f*

veg

This is the best meat-free burger I've ever had. The chickpeas make it rich and satisfying, while the other ingredients give it subtle and surprising flavors. Burger, anyone?

Serves 6

3	cups chickpeas (1 large can), drained
1/2	cup quick oats
1/2	cup green olives or dill pickles, chopped
1	carrot, diced small and blanched
2	tablespoons scallions, thinly sliced
1	level tablespoon white (mild) miso
2	tablespoons soy sauce or tamari
2	teaspoons mustard
2	teaspoons maple syrup
	Cornmeal and 1/2 teaspoon sea salt, for dredging
	Safflower oil

1. In a large bowl, mash chickpeas with a potato masher. Mix in oats, olives or pickles, diced carrot, and scallions. In a separate bowl, blend together miso, soy sauce (or tamari), mustard, and maple syrup and add the blend to the chickpea mixture. Form the mixture into palm-sized patties and dredge them in cornmeal and salt.

2. Heat 3 tablespoons of safflower oil over medium heat. Fry each patty on both sides for 5 minutes. When oil is gone, re-oil the pan for the next round of patties. Serve on whole wheat buns, with toppings, or alone.

P.S.: This mixture freezes well for later use.

continued on next page

* GLUTEN-FREE IF YOU USE TAMARI AND GLUTEN-FREE MISO.

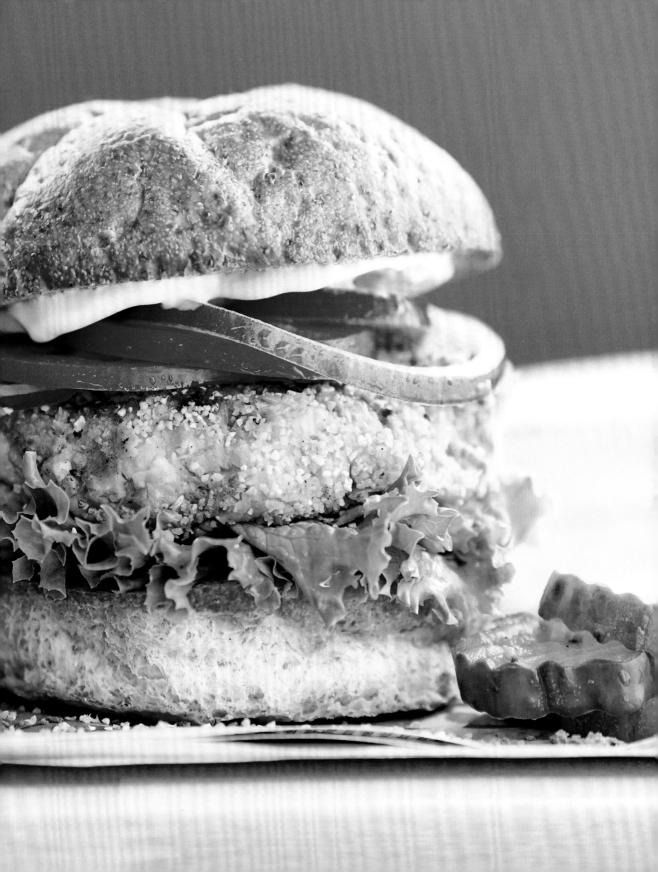

Are Oats Gluten-Free? Technically, yes. But they are often processed in factories that also handle wheat, barley, and other grains that contain gluten, which often contaminate the oats. For people who have celiac disease or who are gluten-intolerant, it can take only trace amounts of the stuff to set off symptoms, so it's best to buy oats that are specifically labeled "gluten-free." That means the supplier has intentionally kept the oats separate from other grains. One more thing: Some gluten-intolerant individuals are also sensitive to oats, regardless of any gluten contamination, so be sure to ask gluten-free friends if they fall into this category before serving them those oatmeal cookies!

TEMPEH BURRITOS

Tempeh is a traditional food from Indonesia. It's made from soybeans that have been fermented, but unless you make it at home, it's going to be pasteurized, so your critters won't get all the benefits of that fermentation. No worries; it's still a rich and satisfying source of plant protein—and totally delicious. Tempeh should always be steamed or boiled for 20 minutes before you do anything else with it; that makes it nice and digestible.

Makes 2 big burritos
or 4 small ones

2	cups water
1/2	cup soy sauce or tamari
1/2	teaspoon brown rice vinegar
1	8-ounce package of tempeh
	Extra-virgin olive oil
1	small onion, diced
	Pinch of sea salt
1/2	teaspoon chili powder
1/2	teaspoon garlic powder
	Whole wheat tortillas
	Tofu Sour Cream (see recipe on page 163)
	Daiya non-dairy cheese shreds
	Shredded lettuce
	Chopped tomatoes
	Guacamole (optional)

I. Combine water, soy sauce (or tamari), and brown rice vinegar and bring to a boil. Cut tempeh into four chunks and add it to the mixture. Let simmer 20 minutes. Set aside.

2. Meanwhile, over medium heat, coat a skillet generously with oil. Sauté the onion with the salt until it becomes translucent. Remove the cooked tempeh from the liquid (save the liquid for later seasoning, if necessary), crumble it into bits like ground beef, and sauté it with the onion.

continued on next page

* GLUTEN-FREE IF YOU USE TAMARI.

Stir in the chili powder and garlic powder. Allow the whole concoction to cook for about 5 minutes. The tempeh should absorb lots of the oil and may even get a little crispy.

3.   Warm a tortilla in another skillet and transfer to a plate. Spread Tofu Sour Cream on the tortilla and add the "beef" (tempeh), cheese shreds, lettuce, and tomatoes, as desired. Wrap the tortilla around the fillings and serve with more sour cream and/or guacamole.

TOFU SOUR CREAM

Makes 2 cups

14 ounces	medium or firm tofu (1 block)
6	tablespoons extra-virgin olive oil
2	tablespoons fresh lemon juice
2	scallions, white parts only
1/2 to 1	teaspoon sea salt

1. Blend tofu, oil, lemon juice, and scallions with 1/2 a teaspoon of salt in a blender or food processor. Taste and add remaining salt, if desired. Serve with burritos, tacos, or any other dish that needs a creamy kick.

Salads
and
Veggies

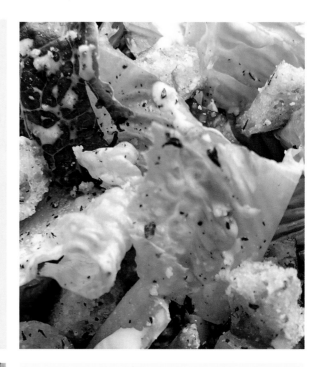

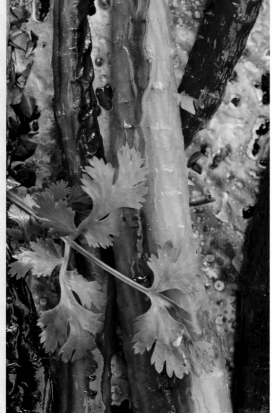

Vegetables are your new best friends, so have fun with these recipes. Did you know that carrots can transform into fettuccine? Or that when you double-bake them, sweet potatoes taste twice as nice? Welcome to a non-dairy Caesar salad and a couple of special seaweed dishes. You will love them!

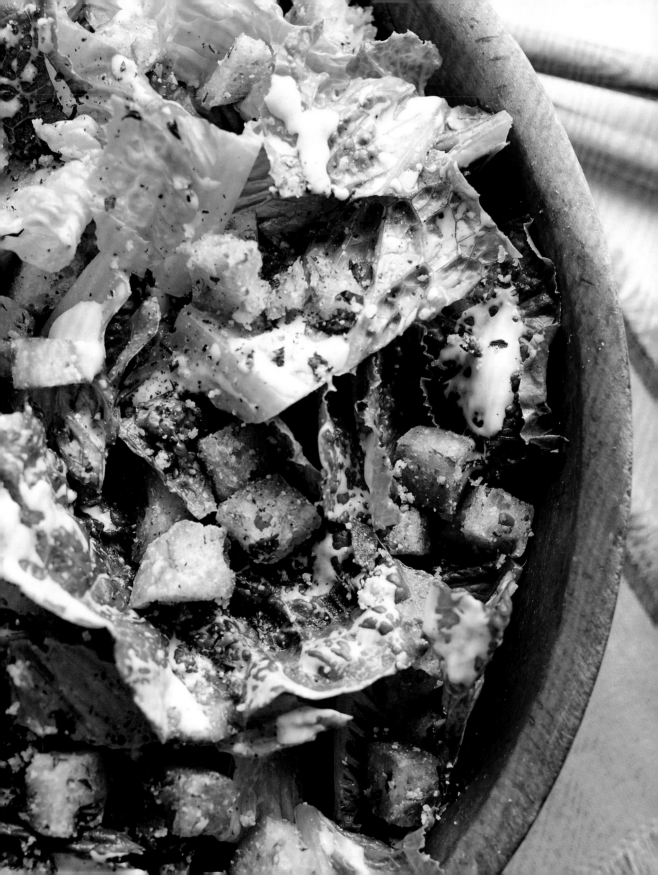

CAESAR SALAD

g-f * Caesar salad is one of my favorites, but after I started my healing process, the cheese no longer worked for me. And then I found dairy-free Parmesan!!! Now I can serve a fantastic Caesar salad to family and friends and no one knows the difference.

Serves 4

FOR THE CROUTONS:

1/2	loaf of baguette, cut into 1/2-inch cubes
	Handful of fresh flat-leaf parsley, chopped
1	tablespoon Non-Dairy Parmesan "Cheese" (page 229)
1	tablespoon extra-virgin olive oil
1/4	teaspoon sea salt
	Freshly ground black pepper to taste

FOR THE SALAD:

1/2	cup regular or vegan mayonnaise
1	garlic clove
	Freshly squeezed juice of 1 lemon
2	splashes of soy sauce or tamari
1	teaspoon anchovy paste
2	tablespoons Non-Dairy Parmesan "Cheese" (page 229)
1/2	teaspoon Dijon mustard
2	romaine hearts, chopped

1. To make the croutons: Add the baguette, parsley, Parmesan, oil, salt, and pepper to a deep bowl. Toss until the cubes are well coated.

2. Heat a 10-inch skillet over medium-high heat. Add the seasoned bread cubes. Cook, shaking the pan every couple of minutes, until the bread is golden and toasted all around. Remove the pan from the heat and set aside.

continued on next page

* GLUTEN-FREE IF YOU USE GLUTEN-FREE BREAD AND TAMARI.

WHOLE NEW YOU

3.   To make the dressing: Add the mayonnaise, garlic, lemon juice, soy sauce (or tamari), anchovy paste, Parmesan, and mustard to a blender. Blend until the dressing is smooth and creamy.

4.   In a deep bowl, combine the croutons and the lettuce. Add half of the dressing, and toss until well coated. Store the remaining dressing in a covered container in the refrigerator (it will last for up to 1 week). Transfer the salad to a platter, or divide among four plates. Serve immediately.

CREAMED SPINACH

Growing up, my sister and I always hated spinach. I guess mom didn't have full-fat coconut milk on hand! FYI, the potato in this recipe thickens it like flour would, while keeping the recipe gluten-free. Russet potatoes are best because they have a higher starch content than other potatoes.

Serves 4

- 1 tablespoon extra-virgin olive oil
- 1 medium yellow onion, chopped fine
- 2 5-ounce bags baby spinach, washed and patted dry
- Sea salt and freshly ground black pepper to taste
- 1 13.5-ounce can full-fat coconut milk
- 1/4 teaspoon freshly grated nutmeg
- 1 small russet potato, chopped fine

1. In a 10-inch skillet, heat the oil over medium heat until shimmering. Add the onion. Cook until lightly golden, 2 to 3 minutes.

2. Add the spinach to the skillet. Season with salt and pepper. Stir in the coconut milk, and add the nutmeg. Add the potato to the pan. Bring to a gentle boil. Reduce heat to low. Cook, stirring occasionally until the sauce has thickened and the coconut milk has reduced by about half, 15 to 20 minutes.

CARROT FETTUCCINE *with* A WARM SHALLOT SAUCE

g-f

veg

The humble carrot is an amazing food, really: full of fiber, complex carbs, vitamins, and antioxidants. It is also sweeeeeeet. When I was detoxing, I found that carrots could satisfy a sweet craving, especially when I chewed them well. This dish is a lovely play on noodles.

Serves 4

10	carrots, scrubbed clean
6	tablespoons extra-virgin olive oil
2	shallots, thinly sliced
2	teaspoons Dijon mustard
1	tablespoon agave syrup
	Sea salt to taste
	Handful of fresh flat-leaf parsley, chopped

1. Prepare the carrots first. Using a vegetable peeler, create ribbons by using a downward motion from the top root of the carrot to the tip; set aside.

2. In a 10-inch deep skillet, heat the oil over medium-high heat until shimmering. Add the shallots. Cook, stirring every couple of minutes so they don't stick to the pan, until well browned and a bit crispy. Using a fork, whisk in the mustard and agave syrup until well blended. Season with salt. Remove the pan from the heat.

3. Add the carrot ribbons to the skillet, tossing to coat them with the sauce. Stir in the parsley. Arrange on a platter to serve family style, or ladle into small bowls to serve.

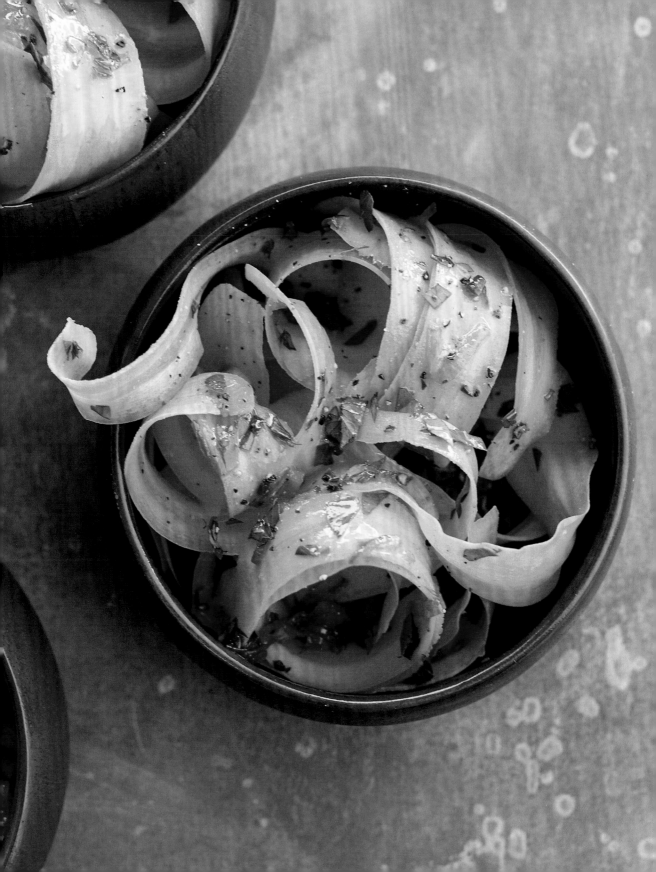

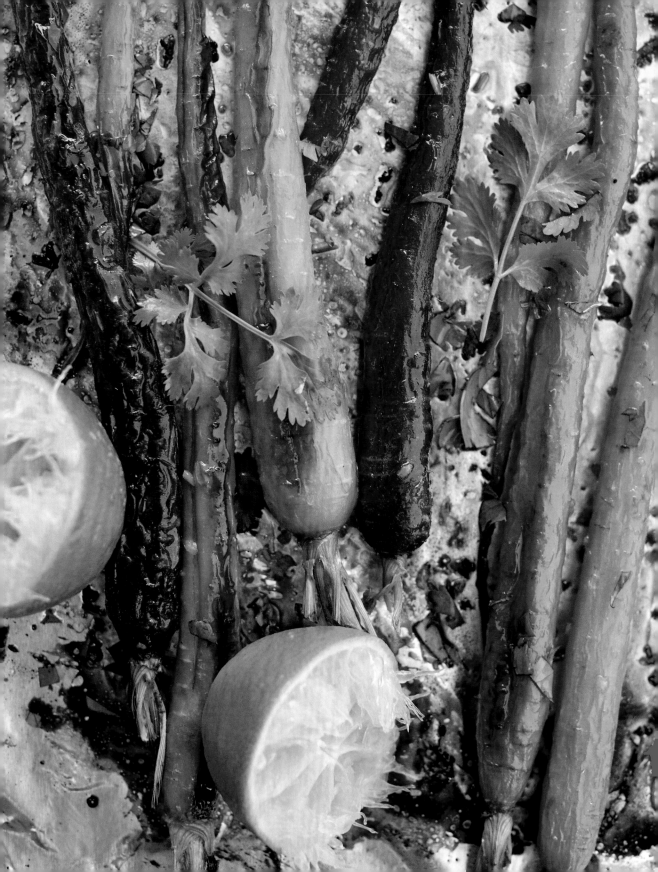

GINGER-LIME ROASTED RAINBOW CARROTS

g-f*

veg

Beautiful. Simple. Mouthwatering. Ladies and gentlemen . . . the roasted carrot!!!

Serves 4

2	tablespoons pure maple syrup
2	tablespoons extra-virgin olive oil
2-inch	piece of fresh ginger, peeled and chopped fine
	Freshly grated zest and juice of 1 lime
1/4	teaspoon sea salt
	Splash of soy sauce or tamari
1	bunch (about 1 1/4 pounds) rainbow carrots, stems trimmed
	Handful of fresh cilantro, chopped (optional)

1. Preheat the oven to 400°F. In a small bowl, combine the syrup, oil, ginger, lime juice and zest, salt, and soy sauce (or tamari). Beat with a fork to mix well.

2. Arrange the carrots in a 9 x 13-inch roasting pan. Pour the syrup-oil mixture over them. Give the pan a few good shakes to coat the carrots. Bake until tender when pierced with a fork, about 1 hour. Garnish with cilantro before serving, if desired. The carrots will taste great served hot, room temperature, and even cold.

To Peel or Not to Peel? When it comes to organic rainbow carrots (which are not only orange, but purple and yellow as well), it's best not to peel. By removing the outer layer, purple carrots lose most of their fantastic color, as many of their cores are orange. Instead, just give them a good wipe or a gentle scrub. Lots of the nutrients are in the skin—or just under the skin—of vegetables, so you're doing yourself a favor by eating them! One exception: Non-organic vegetables are often subject to lots of chemical pesticides and herbicides, so go ahead and peel. Not only will you spare yourself the chemicals, the vegetables will taste better.

* GLUTEN-FREE IF YOU USE TAMARI.

DIJON ROASTED CAULIFLOWER

The modest cauliflower is one of the most delicious foods around. And one of the most versatile: You can steam, roast, or mash it, not to mention throw it into a soup or make it into a pizza crust (page 147)! This delicious recipe shows off the lovely flavor and texture of the 'flower.

Serves 4

1/4 cup extra-virgin olive oil

1 tablespoon mustard (Dijon or whole grain)

1 teaspoon apple cider vinegar

Sea salt to taste

A few splashes of soy sauce or tamari

1 large head of cauliflower (florets only, save stalks for another use)

1. Preheat the oven to 425°F.

2. Add the oil, mustard, vinegar, salt, and soy sauce (or tamari) to a deep bowl. Whisk until well combined. Add the cauliflower. Toss to coat.

3. Spread the cauliflower in a single layer onto an 11 x 17-inch rimmed sheet pan. Bake for 40 to 45 minutes, turning halfway through, until deep golden and tender. May be served immediately, or at room temperature.

Tia Tip: De-flowering cauliflower: When it comes to getting the florets off a head of cauliflower, you have a couple of options: You can definitely get it done with a sharp knife, but I find it's easier to just manhandle them with my bare hands. With some forceful twists, the florets give pretty easily, and I end up getting more cauliflower in the bargain.

* GLUTEN-FREE IF YOU USE TAMARI.

GREEN BEANS & GARLIC SAUCE

g-f*

veg

This dish takes the green bean to a whole new level; between the sesame oil, the soy sauce, and the orange juice, this dish gives the bean a totally revamped personality. And I *love* a vegetable with personality. You will, too!

Serves 4

- 1 tablespoon extra-virgin olive oil
- 1 pound green beans, ends trimmed
- 2 garlic cloves, chopped
- 1/4 cup soy sauce or tamari
- 2 tablespoons sesame oil
- Freshly squeezed juice of 1 orange (about 1/4 cup of juice)
- 1/4 cup vegetable stock
- 1 tablespoon maple syrup
- 2 teaspoons cornstarch
- Red chili pepper flakes (optional)

I. In a 12-inch deep skillet, heat the oil over medium heat until shimmering. Add the green beans. Sauté, uncovered, until slightly tender (crisp to the bite), 8 to 9 minutes. Add the garlic to the pan during the last minute of cooking.

2. Meanwhile, in a small bowl, combine the soy sauce (or tamari), sesame oil, orange juice, stock, syrup, and cornstarch. Whisk until the mixture is well blended and the cornstarch is completely dissolved. Pour the mixture into the skillet, stirring well to coat the green beans. Reduce the heat to medium-low. Cook, stirring occasionally, until the green beans are tender and the sauce has thickened, 3 to 4 minutes more. Top with red chili pepper flakes if desired. Serve hot.

* GLUTEN-FREE IF YOU USE TAMARI.

BAKED SPAGHETTI SQUASH

g-f

veg

clean

I love this dish because it tricks me into thinking I'm having a rich spaghetti dish like the ones I discovered in Italy. It fools the mind into thinking you're eating something that you miss, which is great when you're detoxing.

Serves 2

2   plum tomatoes, chopped

2   garlic cloves, chopped

1   shallot, thinly sliced

4   baby bella mushrooms, chopped
    Sea salt to taste

1   spaghetti squash, cut in half, seeds scooped
    out and discarded

1   tablespoon extra-virgin olive oil (plus more for drizzling)
    Handful of fresh basil, torn

1.   Preheat the oven to 425°F.

2.   In a medium bowl, combine the tomatoes, garlic, shallot, mushrooms, and salt. Stir until well mixed.

3.   Place the spaghetti squash, cut side up, in an 8-inch-square baking pan. Rub the inside of the squash with the oil. Evenly spoon the vegetable filling into the hollowed-out squash. Bake for 45 minutes, until the spaghetti squash easily pulls away from the sides of the skin with a fork. Garnish with the basil before serving.

RED POTATO SALAD

g-f

veg*

clean

God, these potatoes are good—difficult to resist for a kitchen nibbler. And they're even better the next day.

Serves 4

2 large red potatoes, scrubbed clean and cut into 1/2-inch cubes

2 shallots, thinly sliced

1 small red bell pepper, chopped fine

Extra-virgin olive oil, for drizzling

Sea salt and freshly ground black pepper

1/4 cup mayonnaise, vegan mayonnaise, or Aioli (page 121)

1 tablespoon freshly squeezed lemon juice (about 1/2 a lemon)

Handful of fresh dill, chopped

1. Preheat the oven to 425°F. Add the potatoes, shallots, and bell pepper to an 11 x 17-inch rimmed sheet pan. Drizzle 3 to 4 tablespoons of oil over the top. Season with salt and pepper. Use your hands or a rubber spatula to toss everything to combine. Spread the vegetables into a single layer on the pan. Bake for 50 to 60 minutes, stirring halfway through, until the potatoes are deep golden brown and crispy.

2. In a deep bowl, combine the mayonnaise, lemon juice, and dill. Whisk until well combined. Add the still-warm potatoes, shallots, and bell pepper, along with any of the oil and drippings left on the baking sheet. It's important to mix everything while the potatoes are warm, so that they absorb the full flavor of the dressing. Stir until well mixed. The potato salad can be served warm, or you can chill it in the fridge for 1 to 2 days before serving.

* VEGAN IF YOU USE VEGAN MAYO.

SLOW-ROASTED
GRAPE TOMATOES

Mm . . . nothing beats the taste of a great tomato. Except a great *roasted* tomato!

Makes about 1 1/2 cups

2	pints grape tomatoes, cut in half
1/2	cup extra-virgin olive oil
	Sea salt to taste
4	sprigs fresh thyme (leaves only, discard woody stems)

1. Preheat the oven to 250°F. Line an 11 x 17-inch rimmed sheet pan with foil.

2. Arrange the tomatoes in a single layer in the pan. Drizzle the oil over them. Season with the salt and thyme. Give the pan a few shakes until the tomatoes are well coated. Cook for 60 to 75 minutes, until the tomatoes have collapsed slightly and are tender. Serve immediately, or store the tomatoes in a covered container in the fridge for up to 1 week.

SMOKY COLLARD GREENS

g-f

veg

These greens are a spicy version of ones I ate as a kid. I wanted to put my own spin on them because I LOVE HOT SAUCE!

Serves 4

- 1 tablespoon extra-virgin olive oil
- 1 yellow onion, chopped
- 1 bunch collard greens, center ribs removed and leaves chopped
  Sea salt to taste
- 2 teaspoons Spanish paprika
- 2 cups vegetable stock
  Hot sauce to taste (optional)

1. In a 12-inch skillet, heat the oil over medium heat until shimmering. Add the onion. Sauté until golden and tender, 2 to 3 minutes. Add the collards to the pan. Season with salt, and add the paprika. Cook until the collards begin to wilt a little, about 5 minutes.

2. Stir in the vegetable stock. Season with hot sauce, if you are using it. Bring to a boil. Reduce the heat to low, and simmer until the collard greens are very tender and the liquid has reduced by about half, 50 to 60 minutes. Serve hot.

STEAMED VEGETABLES & CURRY SAUCE

We all need to eat our vegetables, and steaming is an easy way to cook them. But steamed vegetables taste even *better* with a lovely sauce. This recipe steams the vegetables in shallow water, but you can also use a steamer over boiling water. Go for it!

Serves 4

1	red bell pepper, seeded and cut into chunks
3	carrots, sliced into 1/4-inch-thick coins
1/2	head broccoli, florets only (save stalks for another use)
1/4	pound green beans, ends trimmed
1	tablespoon coconut oil
2	garlic cloves, grated
2-inch	piece of fresh ginger, grated
1	small yellow onion, grated
2	tablespoons curry powder
1	tablespoon double-concentrated tomato paste
3/4 to 1	cup canned coconut milk
1/2 to 1	teaspoon cayenne (optional)
1	teaspoon freshly squeezed lime juice
	Sea salt to taste

1. Add 1 inch of water to a 2-quart pot. Bring to a boil over high heat. Add the bell pepper, carrots, broccoli, and green beans. Cover tightly with a lid. Cook until the vegetables are tender but still have some bite, about 3 minutes.

2. Then prepare the curry sauce. In a 10-inch skillet, heat the coconut oil over medium heat. Add the garlic, ginger, and onion. Sauté until lightly golden and fragrant, 1 to 2 minutes. Add the curry powder and tomato paste to the pan. Stir until well mixed. Whisk in 3/4 cup of coconut milk, the cayenne pepper (if desired), lime juice, and salt. If you prefer a thinner sauce, stir in the remaining 1/4 cup of coconut milk. Reduce heat to low and simmer for 5 minutes, stirring occasionally.

3. Using a slotted spoon to remove the vegetables from the pot, divide them among four bowls. Spoon the curry sauce on top. Serve immediately.

STUFFED PORTOBELLO
MUSHROOMS

g-f*

veg

clean

These are yummy. I enjoy the meaty taste of the portobellos and the heartiness of the stuffing.

Serves 4

1	cup uncooked millet
	Sea salt to taste
4	portobello mushrooms
2	teaspoons extra-virgin olive oil (plus more as needed)
2	shallots, chopped
1/2	red bell pepper, chopped
	Freshly ground black pepper
1/4	teaspoon cumin
	Splash of soy sauce or tamari
1/2 to 3/4	cup vegetable stock
	Fresh chopped flat-leaf parsley, for garnish

1. Add the millet, salt, and 1 3/4 cups of water to a medium pot. Bring to a boil over high heat. Reduce heat to low. Cook, covered, until all of the water has been absorbed and the millet is tender, about 20 minutes.

2. Meanwhile, preheat the oven to 375°F.

3. Wipe the mushrooms clean. Carefully cut off the stems, and set aside. Use a spoon to scoop out and discard the brown filling inside of the mushroom caps. Arrange the caps in an 8-inch-square baking pan; set aside. Chop the mushroom stems.

4. In a 10-inch skillet, heat the olive oil over medium heat until shimmering. Add the shallots, bell pepper, and mushroom stems to the pan. Season with salt and pepper. Sauté until the shallots and pepper are tender, and the mushrooms lightly golden, 5 to 7 minutes.

* GLUTEN-FREE IF YOU USE TAMARI.

5.   Add the cooked millet, cumin, and soy sauce (or tamari) to the skillet. Give everything a good stir to combine. Stir in 1/2 cup of the stock. If the filling looks too dry, stir in the remaining 1/4 cup of stock.

6.   Rub the mushroom caps with a bit of additional olive oil. Spoon an even amount of filling into each cap, making sure to pat it down. Bake 35 minutes, until the mushroom is very tender. Garnish with parsley before serving.

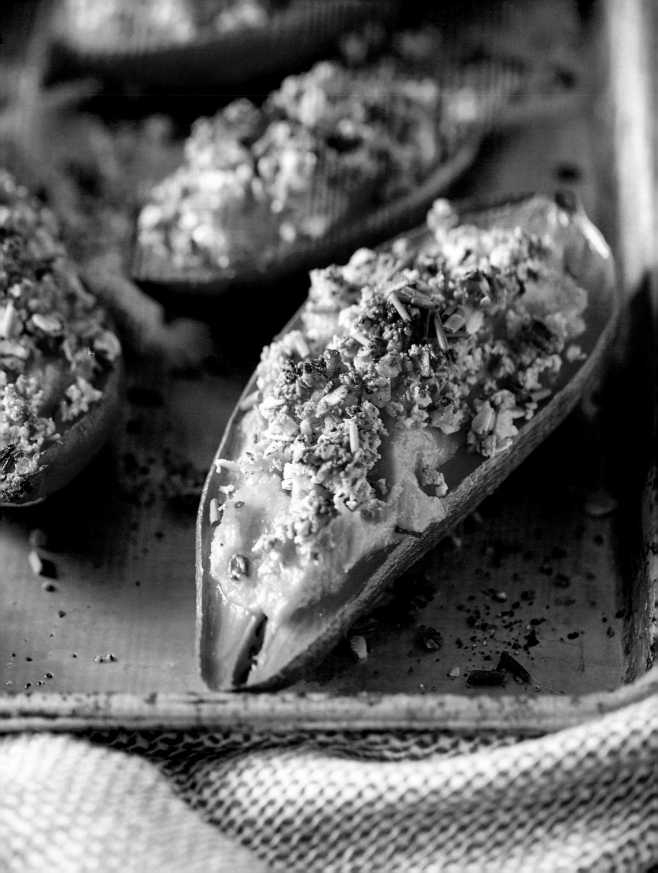

TWICE-BAKED SWEET POTATOES

g-f*

veg

Sweet potatoes are awesome on their own. But if you're like me, you like to make good things even better. Ever mixed cream cheese and coconut cream into a sweet potato and baked it twice? Well, you will now. You're welcome!

Serves 4

FOR THE FILLING:

2	sweet potatoes (12 ounces each), scrubbed clean
1/4	cup unsweetened coconut cream
2	tablespoons dairy-free cream cheese
2	teaspoons chopped chives
1/2	teaspoon sea salt
	Generous pinch of freshly grated nutmeg

FOR THE TOPPING:

1/4	cup walnuts
1/4	cup old-fashioned oats (not quick cooking)
1	tablespoon pure maple syrup

1. Preheat the oven to 400°F.

2. Use a sharp paring knife to make a few slashes all over the sweet potatoes. Place them in an 8 x 8 x 2-inch pan. Bake until very tender when pierced with a fork, 45 to 50 minutes. Remove from the oven, and let cool slightly.

3. Slice the potatoes in half. Use a spoon to scoop the flesh out, making sure to leave a 1/4-inch border inside the potato skins so that they hold their shape. Place the skins back into the baking pan.

4. In a medium bowl, combine the sweet potato filling, coconut cream, cream cheese, 1 teaspoon of the chives, salt, and nutmeg. Use a hand or stand mixer to beat the potatoes until they are well mixed and fluffy. Spoon the filling back into the skins.

continued on next page

WHOLE NEW YOU

5.   To make the topping, add the walnuts and oats to a mini food chopper or food processor. Pulse a few times until coarsely chopped. Stir in the maple syrup. Sprinkle the topping evenly over the filled potato skins.

6.   Bake until the filling puffs up and the topping is golden, 25 to 30 minutes. Garnish with the remaining chives before serving.

CUCUMBER, WAKAME SEAWEED, & RED PEPPER SALAD

g-f

veg

clean

This is one of my favorite ways to consume seaweed; it's light and refreshing and it goes down easy. I got this recipe straight from *The Body Ecology Diet*.

Serves 6 to 8

1/2	ounce wakame flakes
4	large cucumbers, peeled and very thinly sliced
2	teaspoons sea salt or Herbamare
1	large red pepper, diced
1	small red onion, finely chopped
1/3	cup raw, organic apple cider vinegar
2	tablespoons organic, unrefined oil
	Pinch of pepper

1.   Soak wakame for 15 minutes, in enough water to cover it. Sprinkle Herbamare or sea salt on cucumbers and let them sit for several minutes to release their juices. Remove the stem from the wakame and discard the soaking water. Chop the wakame and add it to the cucumbers. Add the diced red pepper and red onion to the cucumbers and wakame. Toss in vinegar, oil, and pepper.

HIJIKI SEAWEED *with* ONIONS & CARROTS

g-f*

veg

clean

Sea vegetables will make your hair, skin, and nails healthy and beautiful. Plus, they will strengthen your bones. Make this dish (or a version of it) once a week, and eat it over two meals. I love seaweed, and I think you'll like it, too!

Serves 4

Small handful dried hijiki (about ⅛ of 2.1-ounce package), soaked in spring water for 30 minutes

2 tablespoons toasted sesame oil

1 onion, sliced in thin half-moons

Pinch of sea salt

1 tablespoon soy sauce or tamari

1 medium carrot, sliced in matchsticks

Corn kernels, from one cob

Scallions, sliced, for garnish

1. While the hijiki is soaking in spring water, chop the vegetables. When the hijiki is soft (after about 30 minutes), discard the soaking water. If the hijiki is in long strands, chop it into 1-inch pieces.

2. Heat the sesame oil over medium heat in a heavy skillet. Add the onion and sauté for a few minutes, adding a pinch of salt. Add the hijiki and sauté it with the onion, coating them lightly in oil. Add water to half-cover the hijiki-onion mixture. Bring to a boil and add soy sauce (or tamari). Cover and let simmer on low for 20 minutes, checking after 10 minutes to make sure it doesn't burn. Most of the liquid should cook off but not to the point of dryness or burning, so add drops of water if needed. Top with carrot matchsticks and corn. Let simmer 10 more minutes. Garnish with scallions.

* GLUTEN-FREE IF YOU USE TAMARI.

BUCKWHEAT STUFFED PEPPERS

g-f

veg

clean

This recipe also comes from *The Body Ecology Diet.* Although it's super clean and healthy, the combination of flavors, textures, and the stuffing of the peppers makes it feel sophisticated and fun.

Serves 6

1	medium onion, chopped fine
1 to 2	tablespoons organic, unrefined coconut oil
1	teaspoon sea salt, or to taste
3/4	teaspoon pepper
2	tablespoons dried sweet basil
2	tablespoons paprika
4 to 6	cloves garlic, chopped fine
2	stalks celery, chopped fine
1	pound greens (e.g., kale), parboiled 5 minutes, chopped
2	cups cooked buckwheat (or quinoa)
6	red peppers, seeded and parboiled 5 minutes

1. Preheat oven to 350°F.

2. Sauté onion in oil with salt, pepper, basil, and paprika until translucent. Add garlic, celery, and greens; cook until tender. Blend with cooked grains. Taste mixture and adjust seasonings. Stuff red peppers with grain mixture. Bake in oiled casserole dish for 45 minutes.

BASIC BUCKWHEAT RECIPE

Serves 4

1 cup buckwheat

2 cups water

Pinch of sea salt

---

1. Soak and rinse buckwheat in a strainer. Place water and salt in a 2-quart saucepan and bring to a rapid boil. Add buckwheat, reduce heat, cover, and simmer until all the water is absorbed (approximately 15 minutes).

Variation: For a rich, nutty flavor, toast the buckwheat (with or without organic, unrefined coconut oil) in a skillet, stirring constantly, before adding it to the water.

ROASTED BEET SALAD

I. Love. This. Dish. First, roasted beets are sweet and sexy. Second, the dressing is elegant and interesting. Third, the quinoa complements both the beets and the dressing beautifully. You cannot go wrong with this recipe.

Serves 4

FOR THE BEETS:

4	red beets, scrubbed
1	tablespoon extra-virgin olive oil
1/2	teaspoon sea salt
1/4	teaspoon black pepper
1	tablespoon orange juice (from one quarter of an orange, if freshly squeezed)

FOR THE DRESSING:

2	tablespoons orange juice (from half an orange, if freshly squeezed)
	Juice of half a lemon
1	small shallot, chopped
1	teaspoon Dijon mustard
1	teaspoon honey
1/2	teaspoon sea salt
1/4	teaspoon freshly ground pepper
1/4	cup extra-virgin olive oil
1	tablespoon hazelnut oil

FOR THE SALAD:

2	cups baby kale
1	avocado, sliced
1	cup cooked quinoa (see chart on page 199)
2	tangerines, segmented
1/2	cup hazelnuts, toasted and chopped

continued on next page

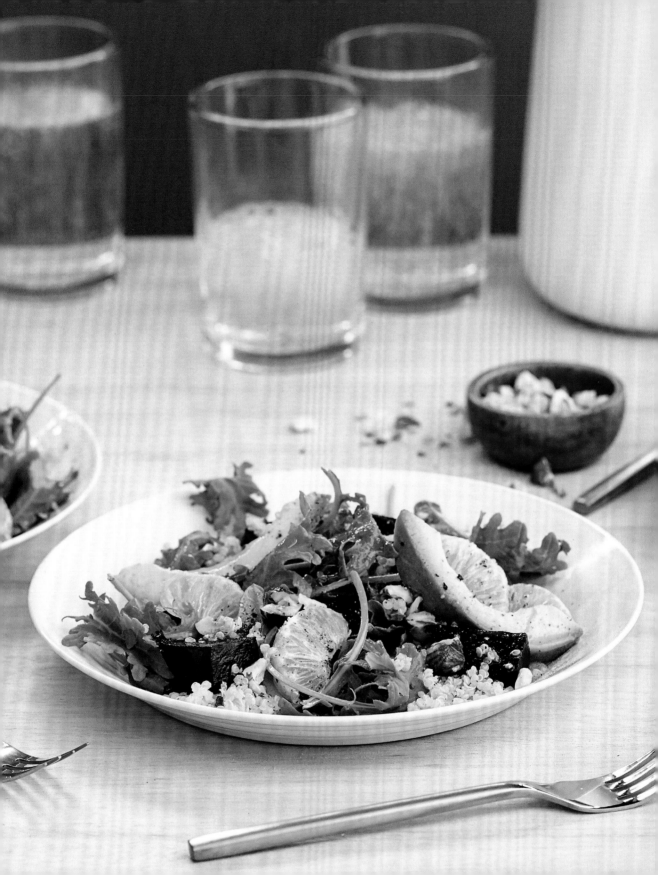

1. To prepare the beets: Preheat oven to 400°F. Toss beets, oil, salt, pepper, and orange juice in a baking dish. Roast for 35 minutes, until the beets are easily pierced with a fork. Remove from oven and let cool. Once cool, skins should easily peel off. Cut beets in quarters and set aside.

2. To prepare the dressing: Combine orange and lemon juices, shallot, mustard, honey, salt, and pepper in a small bowl. Mix well. Slowly add olive and hazelnut oils into dressing, while whisking. Set aside.

3. To assemble the salad: Arrange the kale on a large platter as the base, with each ingredient in separate piles on top of it (the beets will stain the other ingredients). Drizzle with 1/4 cup of dressing and gently toss. Serve.

CRISPY COLLARD CHIPS

When I was on a full cleansing diet, I often had a craving for something bulky, filling, and snacky. So I would make up a big batch of collard or kale chips and feel completely satisfied. The best part was that I never felt guilty, because it was just GREENS! They're a great substitute for potato chips, which may be hard to believe, but when you taste them—with that crunch, and the salty taste—you will become a convert, too.

Serves 4

1   bunch of collard greens, or kale
2   tablespoons extra-virgin olive oil
      Sea salt
1   lemon wedge

1.   Preheat the oven to 275°F. Wash and dry the greens. Cut the stems out and discard, or save for a soup stock. Cut or tear greens into bite-sized pieces. Drizzle the oil and sprinkle a medium-sized pinch of salt over the greens. Massage them until they are well coated with the oil. Place them on a rimmed baking sheet. Bake for 20 minutes and check to make sure that they are crisping up. If you like crispier chips, bake for 10 more minutes. Finish with a squeeze of lemon. Serve.

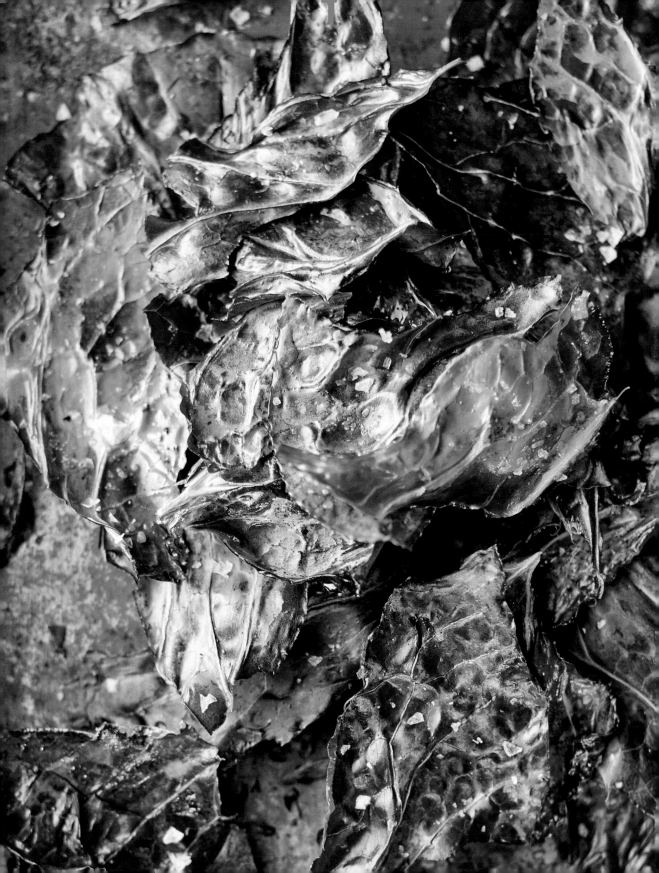

ZUCCHINI *with* SWEET ROASTED KALE & RED ONIONS

g-f

veg

This delicious recipe is by Leslie Bilderback from her book *The Spiralized Kitchen* (St. Martin's, 2015), and you'll need a Spiralizer for it. See page 150 for more information on Spiralizers.

Makes 2 large servings

6 to 8	large kale leaves, stems removed (lacinato—aka Tuscan or dinosaur kale—is best)
1	red onion
3 to 4	tablespoons olive oil
1	cup sliced almonds
3	large zucchini squash
1	clove garlic, minced
	Grated zest and juice of 1 orange
1	tablespoon honey
1	tablespoon balsamic vinegar
1/2	teaspoon kosher salt
1/2	teaspoon white pepper
1/4	teaspoon red chili pepper flakes or more (to taste)

1. Preheat oven to 375°F. Roughly chop the kale, spiralize the onion into thin shreds using the smallest holes, and combine them in a large bowl with 1 tablespoon of olive oil until well coated. Spread onto a baking sheet and roast until the leaves are charred and the onions begin to brown. Spread almonds onto a second baking pan and toast in the same oven until fragrant and golden, about 5 to 10 minutes.

2. Spiralize zucchini into thin shreds using the smallest holes on the Spiralizer. Set aside. Heat 2 tablespoons of olive oil in a large saucepan over medium heat. Add garlic and cook until softened. Stir in orange zest and juice, honey, vinegar, salt, pepper, and chili flakes. Add zucchini and cook, tossing to coat, until just tender, about 2 minutes. Toss in kale and onion just before serving with a garnish of toasted almonds.

Whole Grains and Noodles

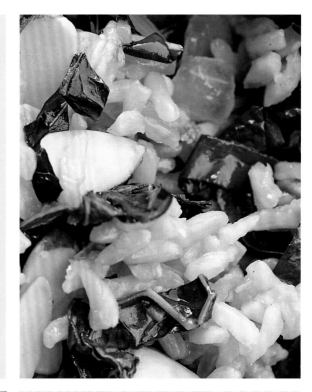

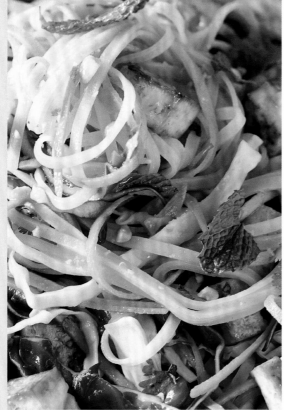

Whole grains provide strong, clean, and stable energy to fuel a fantastic life. In this section, we cover how to cook every major whole grain, and then explore some ideas for dressing them up, deliciously. And we don't stop there: You'll find a few noodle dishes too, to make life just that much nicer.

Cooking
Whole Grains

Most whole grains follow a similar pattern: some version of soak (or roast), boil, salt, and simmer. The differences are in the amount of water used or time cooked. See the chart on the next page.

EQUIPMENT: It's best to cook whole grains in a heavy (or heavy-bottomed) pot, with a heavy, tight-fitting lid. If you don't have one, make sure you cook over a very low flame and find a way to weigh down the lid so it's harder for moisture to escape.

If you're cooking on gas, you can use a flame deflector, or flame tamer, to spread the heat more evenly while the grains are simmering.

Here are the core ingredients in cooking grains:

1   cup grain
    Spring or filtered water
    (see chart for best amount)
    Small pinch of sea salt

1.   Rinse the grain well, discarding any debris. If appropriate, soak the grain for the time mentioned in the chart. Discard soaking water and place grain and measured water in a 2-quart saucepan or other small-to-medium-size pot. Bring to a boil, uncovered. Add the salt, reduce heat to low, and cover with a tight-fitting or heavy lid. Place flame deflector (if you are using one) between pot and flame, and let simmer for appropriate amount of time, undisturbed. When done, remove from heat, and let sit for a minute or two before serving. Some grains, like whole wheat, rye, and spelt, may need to be drained before serving.

GRAIN COOKING CHART

GRAIN	GRAIN-TO-WATER RATIO	SIMMER FOR
MILLET	1:2 TO 3	20 TO 25 MINUTES
QUINOA	1:1.5 TO 2	20 MINUTES
BUCKWHEAT	1:2	15 MINUTES
BROWN RICE *(presoak 3+ hours)*	1:2	50 MINUTES
BARLEY *(presoak 3+ hours)*	1:2	45 MINUTES
SPELT *(presoak 3+ hours)*	1:2	50 MINUTES
RYE *(presoak 3+ hours)*	1:2	50 MINUTES
WHEAT BERRIES *(presoak 3+ hours)*	1:2	50 MINUTES

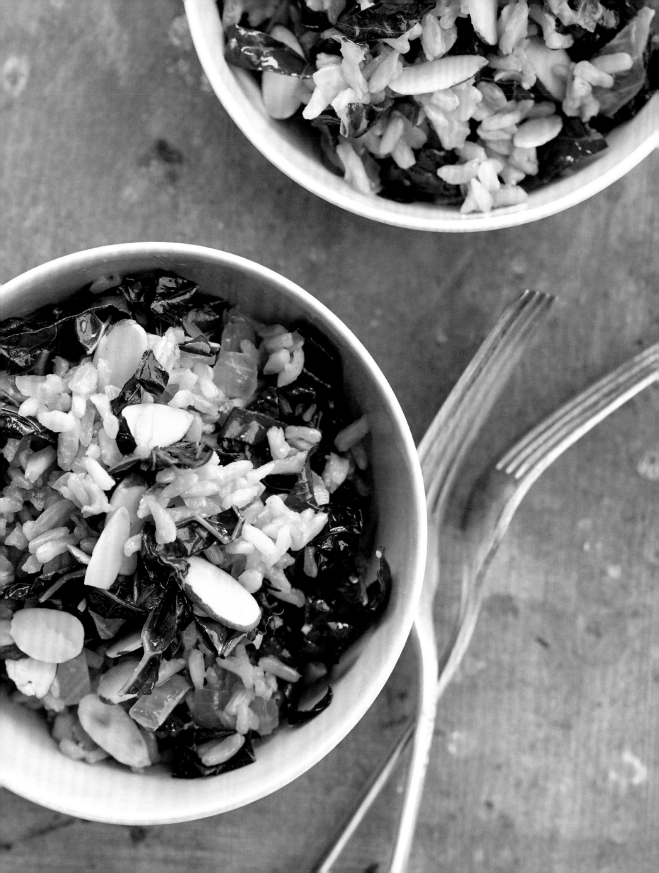

KALE & ALMOND
FRIED RICE

g-f*

veg

clean

This dish combines such interesting tastes and textures, plus it's incredibly good for you. Fried rice, using any combination of vegetables and seasonings, is a wonderful way to sneak whole grains into your family's tummies!

Serves 4

2	teaspoons extra-virgin olive oil
1	medium onion, chopped
1	garlic clove, chopped
1-inch	piece of fresh ginger, peeled and chopped
1/2	bunch Tuscan kale (about 14 leaves), center ribs removed and leaves sliced into ribbons
2	cups cooked, cold brown rice (see Grain Cooking Chart, page 199)
2	tablespoons sesame oil
2	tablespoons soy sauce or tamari
1/4	cup sliced almonds
	Sea salt and freshly ground black pepper to taste

1. In a 10-inch skillet or wok, heat the oil over medium heat. Add the onion, garlic, and ginger. Sauté until lightly golden, 1 to 2 minutes.

2. Add the kale and sauté 2 to 3 minutes, until the leaves are slightly wilted.

3. Add the rice, sesame oil, and soy sauce (or tamari). Cook, stirring frequently, until the rice is heated through. Add the almonds and season with salt and pepper. Serve hot.

* GLUTEN-FREE IF YOU USE TAMARI.

Recently, it was discovered that some rice (even organic brown rice) contains higher-than-normal levels of inorganic arsenic. Even more disturbing amounts were detected in rice products, like rice cereal and brown rice syrup. Over time, too much arsenic can lead to a host of serious health issues, so let's take a look:

Arsenic is a naturally occurring element, present in almost all water and most plants (many of which we eat). There are two types: organic and inorganic (which has nothing to do with pesticide use—these are chemistry terms). Organic arsenic shows up in the tissue of plants, generally through the water that feeds them, and is not really a problem. *Inorganic* arsenic comes from metals found in rocks, and also shows up in industrial pollutants. Too much of this type of arsenic can be dangerous.

So why is rice currently showing higher levels of inorganic arsenic? A couple of reasons: First, rice is a thirsty crop that requires a significant amount of water to grow. If the water being used by the farmer contains inorganic arsenic, the rice will pick it up in greater amounts than many other plants do.

But *where* the rice grows matters, too. Most rice grown in the United States is cultivated in the South (Arkansas, Louisiana, and Texas), and the inorganic arsenic levels in Southern soil tend to be higher than those in California, India, and Pakistan (other rice-growing locales). Why? Well, cotton has been a major crop in the South for more than 300 years, and since the early twentieth century, what did many farmers use as a pesticide for cotton plants? You guessed it: arsenic (technically, the pesticides they used were called "lead arsenate" and "calcium arsenate," but you get the point). So inorganic arsenic has been in Southern soil for more than a hundred years, and the rice plants now growing in those fields are picking it up.

I'm not here to freak you out about rice. Moderate amounts of brown rice are fine, and as a food, rice delivers a huge number of nutritional benefits, in spite of the higher-than-normal levels of arsenic. This is a bigger issue for people who make rice their daily staple grain and eat it in large amounts.

Here's what I suggest:

- Rotate your grains: Make sure to eat quinoa, buckwheat, barley, millet, and other grains in addition to rice. These other grains contain much less arsenic than Southern-grown rice currently does.
- Go easy on rice milks, rice syrup, and rice cereals, and rotate them with other grain-based products. This is especially important for kids.
- Rinse rice well before cooking it.
- If possible, buy rice grown in California.

SOBA NOODLE SALAD

veg This salad is light and refreshing, with an awesome Japanese flair. Although whole buckwheat does not contain gluten, most soba noodles are not 100 percent buckwheat, so this dish does have gluten. In order to make it gluten-free, use rice noodles.

Serves 4

2	tablespoons almond butter
	Freshly squeezed juice of 2 limes
1	tablespoon sesame oil
2	tablespoons soy sauce or tamari
1	teaspoon maple syrup
1	tablespoon extra-virgin olive oil
1/4 to 1/2	teaspoon red chili pepper flakes
1/2	an English cucumber, spiralized (see page 150 for information about spiralizing)
1	large carrot, spiralized
1	red bell pepper, seeded and cut into thin strips
8	ounces soba noodles (prepared according to the package directions)
	Handful fresh chopped cilantro, for garnish
1/2	bunch scallions, chopped, for garnish (white and green parts)
4	teaspoons toasted and sliced almonds, for garnish
4	lime wedges, for garnish

1. In a large bowl, combine the almond butter, lime juice, sesame oil, soy sauce (or tamari), maple syrup, oil, and red chili pepper flakes. Whisk until smooth and well combined. Add the cucumber, carrot, bell pepper, and soba noodles. Toss until the salad is well mixed and coated with the dressing.

2. Arrange the salad on a large platter. Sprinkle the cilantro, scallions, and almonds over the top. Arrange the lime wedges on the platter, and squeeze on top before serving.

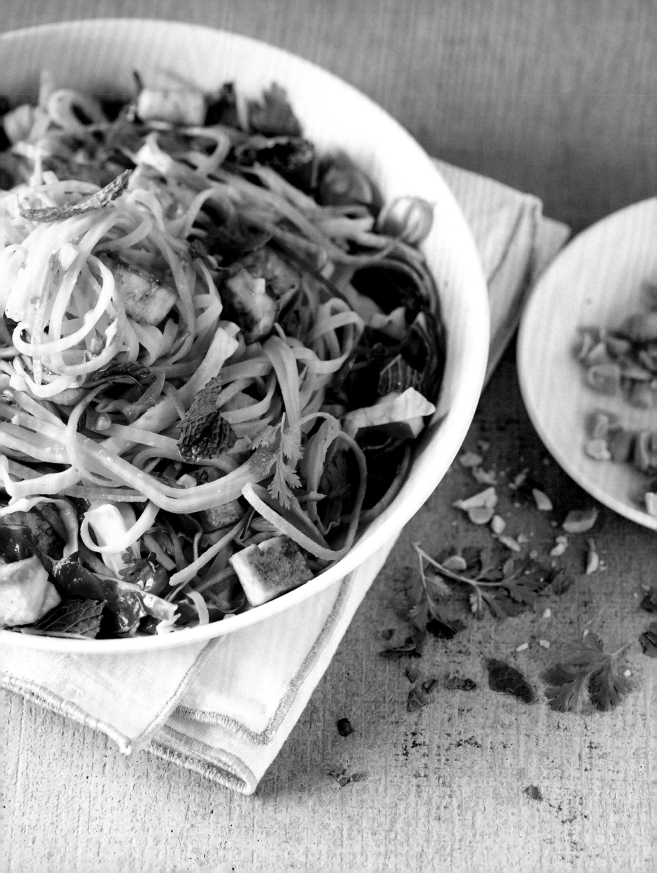

VIETNAMESE RICE NOODLE SALAD

g-f*

veg†

This is a lovely, fresh dish that should be served the day it's made, but the tofu and the dressing can be prepared up to two days in advance. It's also okay to let the salad sit in the fridge for a few hours before serving so that the flavors can meld.

Serves 6 to 8

FOR THE OVEN-FRIED TOFU:

2	tablespoons safflower oil
1	tablespoon soy sauce or tamari
	Splash of mirin (rice wine, available at Whole Foods or Asian markets)
1/2	teaspoon cayenne
	Sea salt and freshly ground black pepper to taste
10	ounces extra-firm tofu, cut into 1/2-inch cubes

FOR THE DRESSING:

	Freshly squeezed juice of 4 limes
1/4	cup extra-virgin olive oil
3	tablespoons brown rice syrup
3	tablespoons brown rice vinegar
3	tablespoons fish sauce (Red Boat brand has no sugar)
1	garlic clove
1	small jalapeño pepper, chopped

FOR THE SALAD:

2	cups thinly sliced green cabbage (about one quarter of a small head)
2	cups thinly sliced red cabbage (about one quarter of a small head)
2	carrots, peeled and shredded
	Handful of fresh mint, torn

continued on next page

* GLUTEN-FREE IF YOU USE TAMARI.

† VEGAN IF YOU SKIP THE FISH SAUCE.

Handful of fresh cilantro, torn

4 ounces brown rice noodles, prepared according to package directions

1/2 cup peanuts, toasted and roughly chopped

I. Preheat the oven to 425°F. Line a baking sheet with parchment paper; set aside.

2. Prepare the tofu: In a medium bowl, combine the oil, soy sauce (or tamari), mirin, cayenne, salt, and pepper. Whisk until well blended. Add the tofu and toss to coat well. Spread the tofu into a single layer on the prepared baking sheet. Bake for 30 minutes, turning halfway through, until deep golden.

3. Make the dressing: In a blender bowl, combine the lime juice, oil, syrup, vinegar, fish sauce, garlic, and jalapeño. Blend until the jalapeño and garlic are fully chopped, and the dressing is well mixed.

4. Assemble the salad: In a deep bowl, combine the cooked tofu, cabbages, carrots, mint, cilantro, and noodles. Pour the dressing over these ingredients and toss until everything is well mixed. Transfer the salad to a serving platter, or divide among individual bowls. Garnish with the peanuts to serve.

Tia Tip: Layer the ingredients of this noodle salad in a Mason jar, with the dressing on the bottom. Take it to work (upright) and shake well before serving. The dressing is also delicious on whole grains or leafy greens.

BARLEY SALAD

veg

clean

This lovely summer salad makes me feel like I'm lunching under the sun in Italy or Spain. Barley, by the way, is great for the skin and is a natural tonic for the liver and gallbladder.

Serves 4

1	cup whole (also known as "hulled") barley
2 1/2	cups water
1	bay leaf
1/2	teaspoon sea salt
7	oil-packed sun-dried tomatoes, diced
3	cloves garlic, minced
2	tablespoons extra-virgin olive oil
1	tablespoon balsamic vinegar
1/2	cup finely chopped cilantro or flat-leaf parsley
1/4	cup Kalamata olives, pitted and quartered lengthwise
1/4	cup toasted pine nuts

1. Bring barley, water, and the bay leaf to a boil in a small saucepan over high heat. When it's boiling, add the salt. Cover, reduce heat to low, and simmer until the barley is tender, about 45 minutes. Drain and cool to room temperature in a bowl.

2. Mix the sun-dried tomatoes, garlic, olive oil, and vinegar, and pour them over the barley. Mix well. Fold in the cilantro, olives, and pine nuts. Cover and refrigerate until cold. Stir before serving.

QUINOA TABBOULEH

I love Middle Eastern food and this is an adaptation of traditional tabbouleh. Thanks to the olives, cucumber, parsley, and lovely dressing, the flavors take me back to my trip to Cairo. Well, Cairo . . . via *Peru*. You see, quinoa is a superfood grown in the Andes of South America. It's high in protein, minerals, and fiber and has a slightly nutty flavor. Global cuisine!

Serves 4 to 6

1	cup quinoa
1 1/2	cups spring water
1/4 to 1/2	teaspoon sea salt
	Peppermint tea bag (optional)
1/4	cup extra-virgin olive oil
2	cloves garlic, minced
1/4 to 1/3	cup lemon juice
1	tablespoon fresh mint, chopped fine
1	small tomato, diced (optional)
1	cup cucumber, diced
1/4	cup kalamata olives, halved
1/4	red onion, sliced finely into half-moons
1/4	cup chopped parsley

1. Rinse quinoa well. Over medium-low heat, dry roast it in a skillet for a few minutes, stirring continually until it gives off a slightly nutty aroma.

2. Bring the water, salt, and, if desired, tea bag to a rolling boil in a small pot. Boil for 1 minute and remove the tea bag. Add the quinoa, cover, and reduce heat to low. Let simmer 20 minutes or until all water is absorbed. Spoon the quinoa into a bowl to cool.

3. Combine the oil, garlic, lemon juice, and mint into a dressing. When the quinoa is cool, toss in the tomato (if you're using it), cucumber, olives, onion, parsley, and dressing to taste. Serve immediately or chill first. Great with pita bread and hummus.

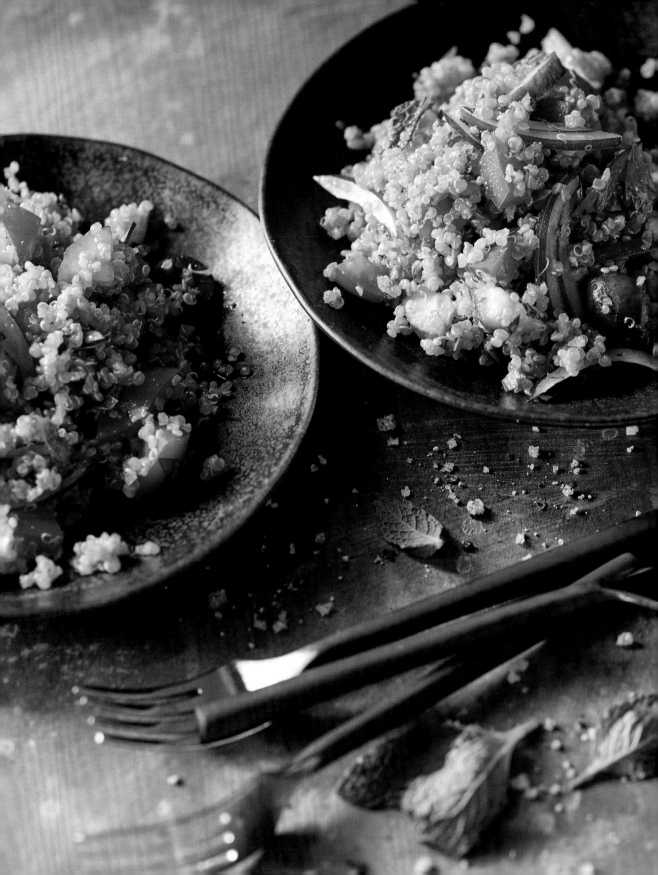

Fermented Foods

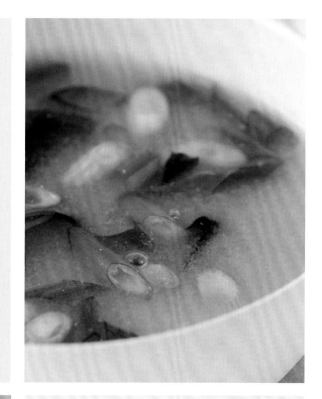

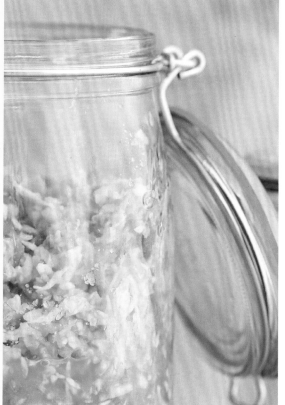

There's no reason to be intimidated by fermented foods: Miso soup is delicious and easy to prepare at home, and pickling or fermenting vegetables is simple and produces super healthy benefits. The following recipes will give you a few approaches, but feel free to supplement them with good-quality unpasteurized pickles or cultured vegetables from a trustworthy health-food store.

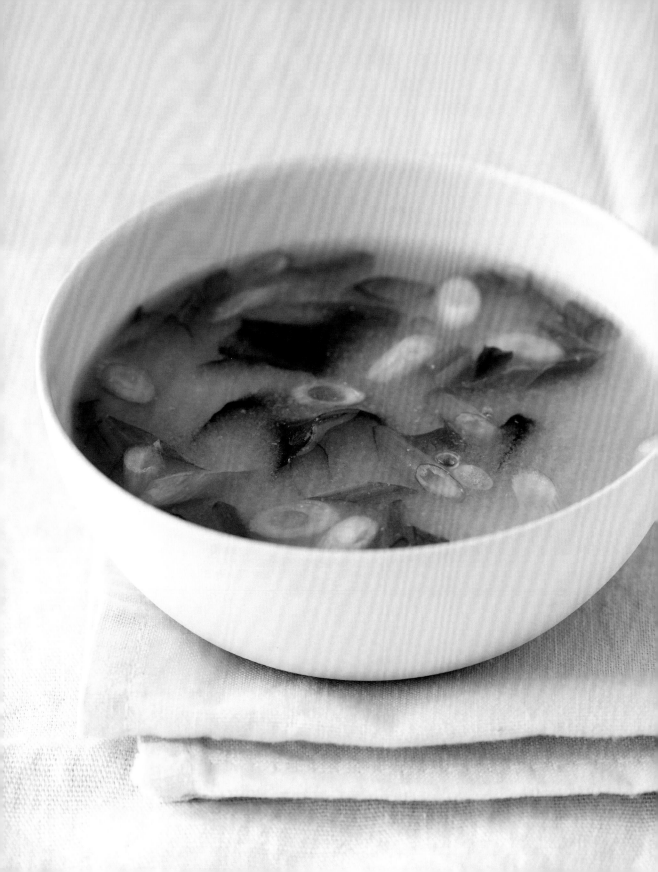

MISO SOUP

Miso's fermentation is what makes it so healthy. In fact, it may be one of the health-iest things you can put in your body; naturally anti-inflammatory, miso blocks tumor growth, discharges toxins, and delivers good-quality gut bacteria. You can't do better than that. In Japan, miso soup is eaten every day, and Japanese people have some of the longest life spans in the world. And did I mention that it's crazy delicious? One rule of thumb: Never use more than one teaspoon of miso per cup of liquid. Too much miso will taste salty and leave you thirsty and craving sweets.

Serves 3

3	cups water
1	2- to 3-inch piece of kombu (dried kelp)
1 1/2	teaspoons wakame flakes
1	tablespoon miso paste (South River Miso or Miso Master are best)
2	tablespoons sliced scallions

1. In a medium saucepan, bring the water and kombu to a boil. Turn the heat down to low and remove the kombu, reserving it for another use. Add the wakame flakes and let them expand.

2. Transfer 1/2 cup of broth to a small bowl and whisk with the miso paste until well blended. Return the miso mixture to the saucepan. Let the soup simmer on very low heat for 3 to 4 min-utes to allow the miso to integrate properly. Miso should never come to a boil; the bacteria will be destroyed.

3. Stir well and serve with scallions.

Variation: You can really go wild with miso soup, using all sorts of vegetables and different types of miso. You can even add fish or tofu! The only things that should remain consistent are the water, miso, and wakame seaweed.

* GLUTEN-FREE IF THE MISO IS GLUTEN-FREE.

CULTURED VEGETABLES

g-f

veg

clean

This is a slight adaption of the recipe from *The Body Ecology Diet.* These cultured vegetables are responsible for strengthening my health and immunity, one bite at a time. I am insanely grateful for that, and I urge you to make this recipe.

One important secret to making really delicious yet medicinal cultured veggies is to use freshly harvested, organic, well-cleaned vegetables. After washing the veggies, spin them dry. Clean equipment is essential. Rinse everything you use in very hot water.

*Makes approximately 12 to 20 servings, depending on the size
of the cabbage and the length of fermentation.*

VERSION 1

1	head cabbage, shredded in a food processor
2	large carrots, shredded in a food processor
1-inch	piece of ginger, peeled and chopped
2	cloves garlic, peeled and chopped

VERSION 2

1	head cabbage, shredded in a food processor
2 to 3	leaves of kale, chopped by hand
2/3	cup wakame sea vegetables, measured after soaking (optional)
1	teaspoon dill seed

1.   Combine all ingredients in a large bowl. Remove about 1 to 2 cups of the mixture and place them in a blender. Add enough filtered water to make a "brine" with the consistency of a thick juice. Blend well and then add the brine back into the main mixture. Stir well.

2.   Pack the mixture into an airtight glass or stainless-steel container. Use your fist, a wooden dowel, or a potato masher to pack the veggies tightly. Fill the container almost full, leaving about 2 inches of room at the top for the veggies to expand. Roll up several cabbage leaves into a tight "log" and place them on top to fill the 2-inch space. Clamp the jar closed.

3.   Let the veggies sit at room temperature for at least three days. A week is even better. You may see vegetables begin to bubble, which is good, and after a week, you can "burp" them, by opening the lid and releasing the pressure inside, if necessary. Refrigerate to slow down fermentation. Enjoy!

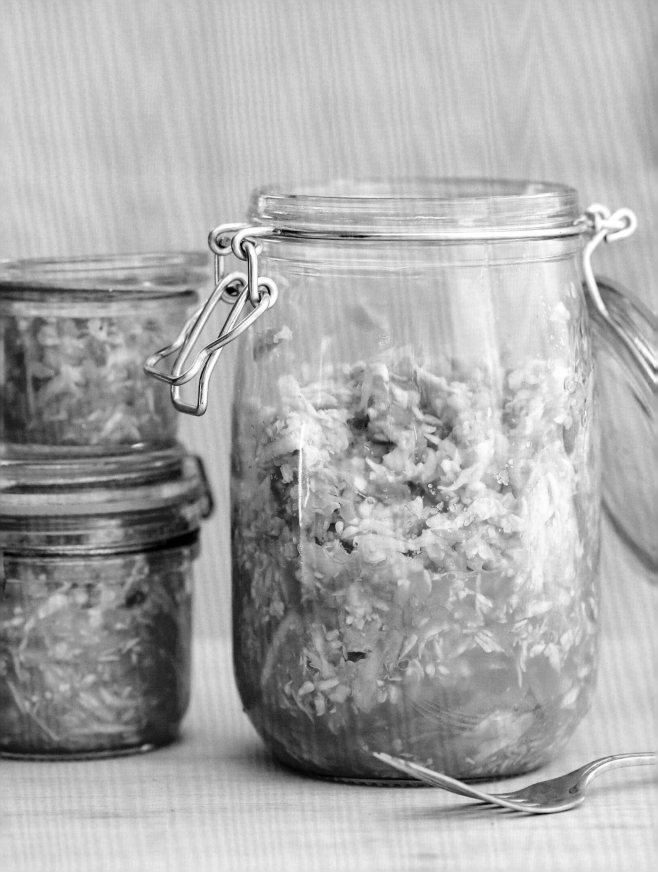

KIMCHI

*g-f**

veg

clean†

When I was little, my family lived in Hawaii for a while. There is a big Korean community there, and I've been eating kimchi ever since. As a kid, I just loved how it tasted, and as an adult, I was thrilled to discover its health benefits. By the way: To get your daily cultured vegetable, you can eat kimchi straight-up, fold it into fried rice, or plunk it on top of a taco or sandwich.

Makes about 1 1/2 quarts

1	medium head (1 1/2 pounds) Napa cabbage, cored and cut into 2-inch strips
8	ounces daikon (Chinese radish), cut into matchsticks
2	tablespoons kosher salt
2-inch	piece of fresh ginger, peeled and grated
6	garlic cloves
2	tablespoons Korean red chili pepper flakes (also called *gochugaru*)
1/2	bunch scallions, chopped (green and white parts)
2	tablespoons miso paste

1. In a deep bowl, combine the cabbage, daikon, and salt. Toss to mix well. Let sit at room temperature, uncovered, for 90 minutes, to draw out some of the water from the cabbage. Drain and rinse under cold water a few times, to wash off most of the salt. Let the cabbage and daikon mixture sit in the strainer for 30 minutes to drain further.

2. Meanwhile, add the ginger, garlic, red chili pepper flakes, scallions, and miso paste to the bowl of a food processor. Pulse until it forms a smooth paste, 1 to 2 minutes.

3. Put on a pair of food-safe rubber gloves (do not skip this step; the Korean pepper flakes are very strong and may burn or discolor your hands). In a large bowl, combine the cabbage, daikon, and chili paste. Rub the mixture together with your hands to really coat the cabbage. Stir in 3/4 cup of water.

4. Fit a funnel over the mouth of a 3 1/2-quart glass jar. Spoon the kimchi into the jar, pressing

* GLUTEN-FREE IF MISO IS GLUTEN-FREE.

† (ALTHOUGH RED CHILI PEPPER FLAKES MAY NOT WORK FOR EVERYONE)

down often to really pack it in. The kimchi is ready to eat immediately, if desired, but is best eaten after the seasonings have had time to mature. Seal the jar closed if you can resist the temptation, and store it in the fridge for 1 week. The kimchi will last up to 2 months in the fridge.

What you need to make Kimchi: 1. An airtight jar. I like Mason jars, but I find that the ones with the flip lids work better than the ones with the screw tops. 2. Thin, food-safe rubber gloves because you will be handling VERY HOT peppers that may burn or discolor your hands. (You can skip the gloves if you skip the peppers.) These gloves can be found online or at major retail stores.

What is daikon? Pronounced "DIE-con," this long white radish was cultivated originally in Southeast and East Asia, but now grows in many places. Milder than a red radish, daikon is pungent when raw but tastes slightly sweet when it's cooked. Daikon is great in soups, stews, and salads and is especially tasty as a pickle. Daikon is low in calories, helps to emulsify fats (you may notice a little mound of grated daikon beside your tempura at a Japanese restaurant), is a natural diuretic, and helps the body break down animal protein (it's also served with sashimi, in raw shreds). Try daikon!

SAUERKRAUT

Turns out that Eastern Europeans have also been feeding their microbiome for centuries! Sauerkraut is remarkably easy to make, and an excellent snack to have in the fridge. After you've done it once, you'll have it down.

Makes about 1 1/2 quarts

1   medium head green cabbage, cored and shredded, with one large outer leaf preserved

1   tablespoon sea salt

1.   In a deep bowl, combine the cabbage and salt. Using your hands, squeeze the cabbage until it becomes slightly limp and wilted and begins to release liquid. Spoon the cabbage into a 4-quart glass jar, constantly pushing it down to pack the cabbage in tightly.

2.   Place the large outer leaf of the cabbage over the shredded cabbage to keep it submerged in the liquid. Rest a smaller glass jar filled with dried beans (or filled with something else that's dry and heavy) on top of the cabbage leaf. The smaller jar will continue to weigh down the mixture as it ferments. Seal the larger jar closed with a lid.

3.   Press down every few hours for the first 24 hours of fermentation. If the cabbage hasn't released enough liquid to cover itself by the end of the first day, mix 1 teaspoon of salt with 1 cup of water and pour just enough of this mixture over the cabbage until it's covered.

4.   Let the jar sit for at least 2 more days in a cool spot, out of direct sunlight. Press the jar down daily at this point. You'll see bubbles form on top and hear a pop when you open the jar—this is normal. You can skim the foam off the top, if you wish.

5.   Begin tasting it on day 3 to see if it's to your liking. You can continue to let it ferment for up to 7 more days in a cool, dark spot (for a total of 10 days fermentation). The sauerkraut should then be refrigerated (remove the jelly jar weighing it down) and eaten within 2 months.

Dressings and Sauces

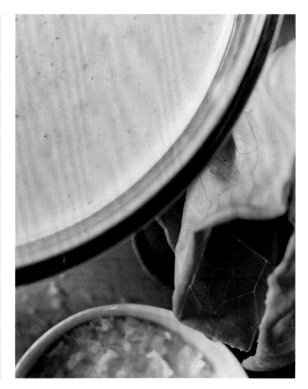

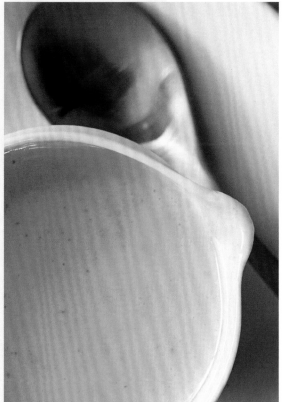

A great dressing or sauce can raise a dish to a whole new level. Whether your favorite is hollandaise on eggs Benedict or a dairy-free ranch on a tossed salad, these recipes will take your cooking up a notch.

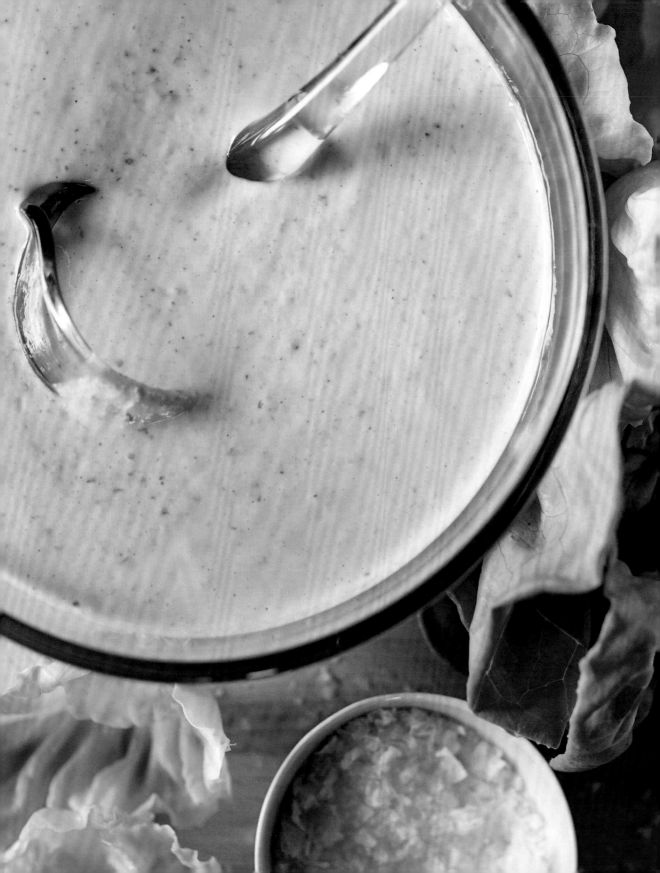

CREAMY RANCH DRESSING

g-f

veg

Sometimes you just need a big dollop of ranch dressing. And this one is super healthy. Enjoy!

Makes 1 1/2 cups

8	ounces silken tofu
1/2	cup vegan mayonnaise
2	tablespoons safflower oil
1	tablespoon apple cider vinegar
1	garlic clove
1	small onion, chopped
	Small handful of fresh flat-leaf parsley
1/4	teaspoon paprika
	Sea salt to taste

1. In a blender bowl, combine the tofu, mayonnaise, oil, vinegar, garlic, onion, parsley, and paprika. Blend until smooth and creamy. Season with salt. Transfer the dressing to a glass jar, cover, and refrigerate for at least 2 hours or up to 1 week. This dressing is fine to use immediately, but I also think it gets better after a day or two in the fridge. Try it and decide for yourself!

CREAMY PUMPKIN DRESSING

g-f

veg

Pumpkin seeds contain tons of magnesium and omega-3 fatty acids, not to mention lots of zinc, which is especially good for men. But that's not all: Pumpkin seeds help to regulate blood sugar, are anti-inflammatory, and might even help you sleep!

Makes 1 ¹/₄ cups

¹/2	cup pumpkin seeds
1	small, very ripe avocado
¹/3	cup freshly squeezed lemon juice (from about 3 lemons)
	Sea salt to taste
	Handful of fresh flat-leaf parsley
¹/2	cup extra-virgin olive oil
	Splash of red wine vinegar

I.   Add the seeds to the bowl of a blender. Pulse until they form a coarse breadcrumb-like texture. Add the avocado, lemon juice, salt, parsley, olive oil, and vinegar. Pulse until the mixture forms a thick, smooth dressing, 1 to 2 minutes. The dressing is ready to use immediately, or may be stored in a tightly sealed jar in the fridge for up to 3 days.

SMOKY BLACK BEAN SAUCE

g-f

veg

This sauce can add a Mexican kick to many dishes: Try it on grains, vegetables, or anything that makes you happy.

Makes 2¹/4 cups

1	15.5-ounce can black beans, including liquid
2	teaspoons extra-virgin olive oil
1/2	red bell pepper, chopped fine
1	small yellow onion, chopped fine
1	garlic clove, chopped fine
	Sea salt to taste
1	cup vegetable stock
2	teaspoons Spanish paprika

1. Add the black beans to the bowl of a food processor. Pulse until they form a chunky purée; set aside.

2. In a 10-inch skillet, heat the oil over medium heat until shimmering. Add the bell pepper, onion, and garlic. Season with salt. Sauté until lightly golden and tender, 2 to 3 minutes.

3. Add the black beans, vegetable stock, and paprika to the skillet. Stir until well mixed. Bring to a boil, then reduce heat to low. Continue to cook, stirring occasionally, until the sauce thickens and reduces by about a third, 8 to 10 minutes. Serve hot.

EASY BLENDER
HOLLANDAISE SAUCE

g-f

Unlike many other sauces, hollandaise needs to be made right before serving. Great for eggs Benedict, drizzled over vegetable dishes, or as a topping on fish.

Makes about 1 cup

3	large egg yolks (save whites for another use)
1	tablespoon freshly squeezed lemon juice (from about 1 lemon)
1/4	teaspoon sea salt
1/8	teaspoon cayenne
6	tablespoons coconut oil, melted

1. In a blender bowl, combine the egg yolks, lemon juice, salt, and cayenne. Cover and blend until well combined, 1 minute.

2. With the blender on medium-high speed, slowly drizzle in the oil a few drops at a time. This should take about 2 minutes, during which time the mixture will begin to thicken. Use immediately.

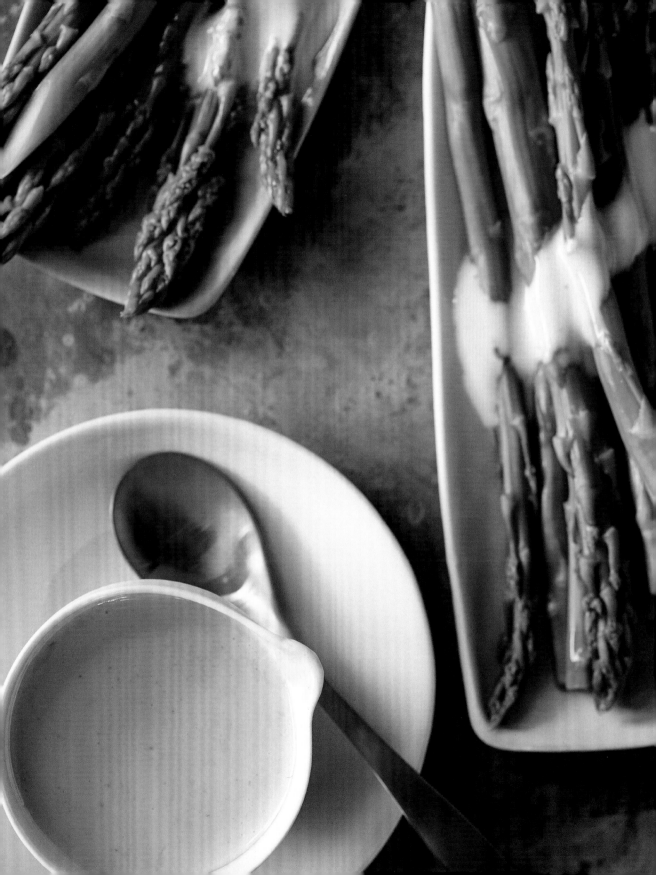

BASIL PESTO

g-f

veg

Fresh basil has such a right-out-of-the-garden-on-a-summer-day taste, and I ate tons of it in Italy. But traditional pesto contains cheese, so I had to find a new way to make it. This recipe uses a dairy-free Parmesan cheese (page 229), which you'll see in a handful of my recipes. There are few options out there on the market, like the Go Veggie brand, but you can also make your own.

Makes 3/4 cup

1/4	cup pine nuts, toasted
2	cups (packed) fresh basil (leaves only)
	Sea salt to taste
	A few grinds of freshly ground black pepper
1/4	cup Non-Dairy Parmesan "Cheese" (page 229)
1/4 to 1/2	cup extra-virgin olive oil

1. Add the nuts to the bowl of a food processor. Pulse until chopped fine. Add the basil, salt, pepper, and Parmesan. Pulse until it forms a paste. Using the feed tube on the food processor, drizzle in 1/4 cup of the olive oil while it's processing. If you prefer a thinner pesto, drizzle in the remaining 1/4 cup of oil. The pesto is ready to use immediately, or may be stored in a covered container in the fridge for up to 1 week.

ROASTED MARINARA SAUCE

This is a delicious marinara sauce, if I do say so myself; the basil, garlic, and onions give it real depth and character. Try it on noodles or grains.

Makes about 3 cups

1	28-ounce can crushed tomatoes
1	large yellow onion, cut in half (through the root)
1	garlic clove, smashed
1/2	teaspoon sea salt (plus more to taste)
	Freshly ground black pepper to taste
	Handful of fresh flat-leaf parsley, chopped, plus more for garnish
8 to 10	fresh basil leaves
2	tablespoons extra-virgin olive oil

1. Preheat the oven to 325°F.

2. Add the tomatoes, onion, garlic, salt, pepper, parsley, basil, and oil to a 4-quart Dutch oven. Stir to combine. Simmer, uncovered, for 1 hour, stirring occasionally. The sauce is ready to serve immediately. Alternately, cool it completely and store it in the fridge in a covered container for up to 3 days, or in the freezer for up to 2 months.

CARROT-GINGER DRESSING

g-f*

veg

This is just like the yummy carrot dressing that's served on fresh salad at Japanese restaurants. My favorite!

Makes 1 cup, which serves 4 to 6

1	tablespoon carrots, minced
1	tablespoon ginger root, peeled and minced
1/3	medium onion, chopped (about 1/3 cup)
1	tablespoon finely chopped lemon (with some rind)
2 1/2	tablespoons soy sauce or tamari
1/4	cup light olive oil
1/4	cup brown rice vinegar
1	tablespoon brown rice syrup
1/4	cup water
2	teaspoons sugar-free ketchup
	Pinch of sea salt (optional)
	Pinch of fresh ground black pepper

1. Blend all ingredients in blender. Serve immediately.

* GLUTEN-FREE IF YOU USE TAMARI.

NON-DAIRY
PARMESAN "CHEESE"

Makes 1 cup

1	cup raw cashews
4	tablespoons nutritional yeast
1	teaspoon sea salt
1/2	teaspoon garlic powder

1. Place all ingredients in a food processor. Blend until well mixed, or until it reaches the desired consistency. Keep in the refrigerator for up to 3 weeks.

What Is Nutritional Yeast? These golden yellow flakes can be found in the bulk section of most health-food stores and are actually a form of *deactivated* yeast, so they are unable to leaven bread or baked goods. Instead, these yummy flakes—often fortified with vitamin B12—give a cheesy taste to popcorn, scrambled tofu, dips, or anything else you want to sprinkle them on. Check them out!

Breakfasts

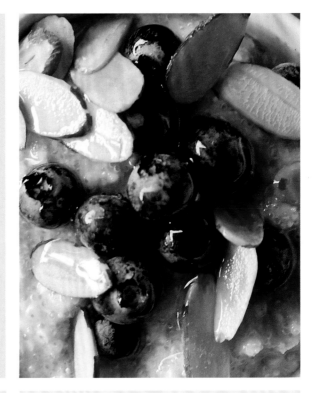

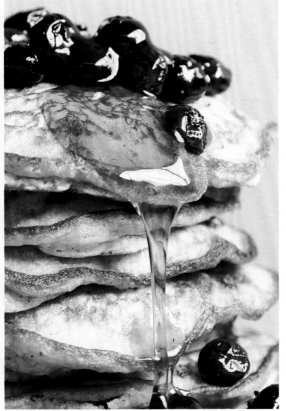

Good morning! I've created a bunch of healthy, lip-smacking breakfast dishes, designed to start your day off right. I presume you already love a good banana pancake or blueberry muffin, but have you ever made them without white sugar and dairy? Well today, my friend, is your lucky day . . . I mean, *morning*!

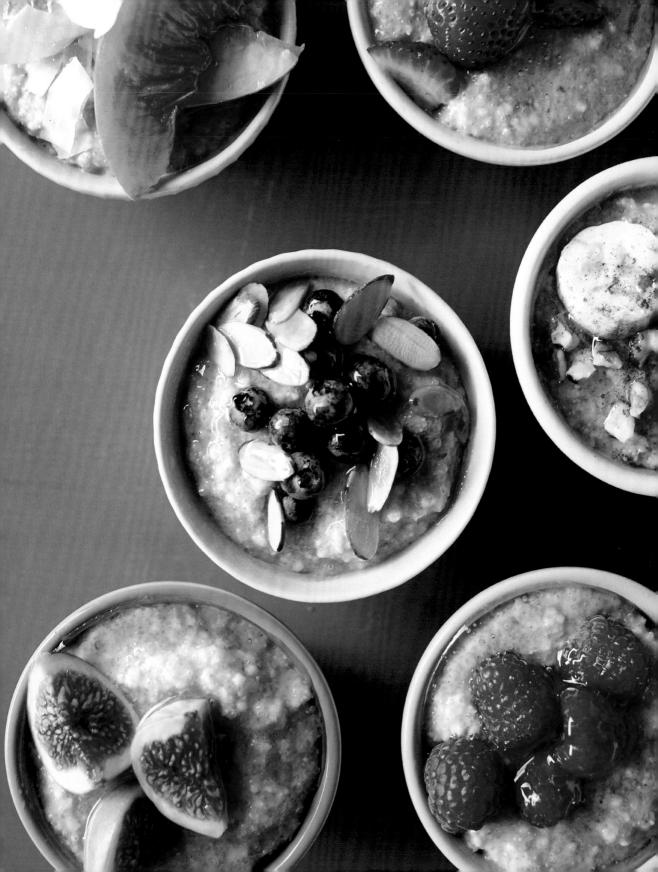

AMARANTH & MILLET PORRIDGE *with* BANANAS, FIGS, & ALMONDS

Millet is a great grain; it's filling, easy to digest, and provides smooth energy. Amaranth, from South America, is a cousin to quinoa and gives this recipe a neat texture and taste.

Serves 4

1/2	cup amaranth
1/2	cup millet
1 3/4	cups boiling water
3/4	cup non-dairy milk of your choice (cashew, almond, coconut, soy)
1	very ripe banana, mashed
8	fresh figs, cut into quarters
1/4	cup sliced almonds, toasted
4	teaspoons maple syrup (optional)

1. In a 2-quart pot, combine the amaranth, millet, and boiling water. Let the mixture soak overnight.

2. In the morning, add the milk to the pot. Bring it to a gentle boil, then reduce the heat to low. Cook for 8 to 10 minutes, until the grains are tender (the amaranth will still have a nutty texture that pops when you eat it).

3. Stir in the mashed banana. Divide the porridge among four bowls. Top with the figs, almonds, and maple syrup, if desired.

Tia Tip: Create a Topping Bar for the kids! Using small bowls or jars, set out a selection of fruits, nuts, seeds, and other toppings so the kids can choose their own. Fun things to try: coconut flakes, goji berries, pomegranate seeds, roasted pumpkin seeds . . . even seaweed powder!

BANANA PANCAKES *with* BLISTERED BLUEBERRIES

 g-f* Did I mention I love pancakes? Well, I still eat them. However, these ones are filling and energizing without leaving me bloated, and they're a fun way to start the morning. They're also a favorite of Cree's—your kids will love 'em, too!

Serves 4

1	cup oat flour
2	teaspoons baking powder
1	teaspoon coconut sugar
1/2	teaspoon sea salt
1/4	teaspoon freshly grated nutmeg
3/4	cup almond milk
1	large egg
1	teaspoon pure vanilla
2	ripe bananas, mashed well
1/2	pint fresh blueberries
	Grapeseed oil to coat the skillet
	Pure maple syrup (optional)

1. In a medium bowl, add the flour, baking powder, coconut sugar, salt, and nutmeg. Whisk to combine.

2. In a separate bowl, add the almond milk, egg, and vanilla. Beat with a fork or whisk until blended. Pour the milk mixture over the flour mixture. Add the mashed bananas. Using a fork, stir until just combined. Let the batter sit for 5 minutes so the baking powder can activate.

3. Meanwhile, add the blueberries to an 8-inch skillet over medium-high heat. Cook, shaking the pan a few times, until the blueberries deepen in color and look like they're about to burst (it's okay if some do), 3 to 4 minutes. Remove from heat, and set aside.

4. Add a few drops of oil to a 10-inch skillet over medium heat. Once the oil is shimmering, drop 1/4 cup of batter at a time into the pan (you'll need to cook the pancakes in 3 to 4 batches).

continued on next page

BREAKFASTS

* CONTAINS GLUTEN UNLESS OAT FLOUR IS MARKED "GLUTEN-FREE."

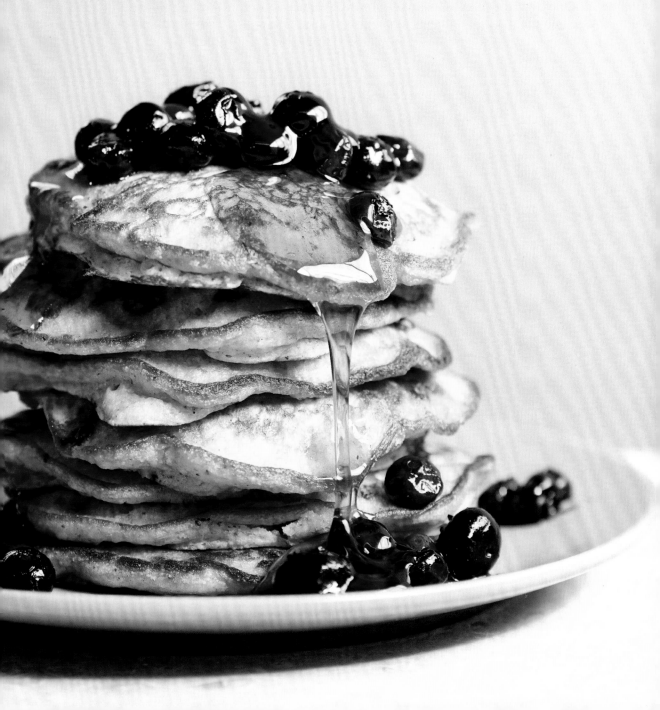

Cook until the edges of the pancakes look set and little air bubbles form on top, about 2 minutes. Then, using a spatula, flip the pancakes and continue cooking for 1 to 2 minutes more until they are golden underneath. Repeat with the remaining batter.

5. To serve, top with some of the blueberries and maple syrup, if desired.

Tia Tip: WHY THE FORK? When mixing muffin and pancake batters, I like to use a fork; it acts like a little rake and helps to scrape up the dry ingredients at the bottom of the bowl, without over-mixing the batter.

BLUEBERRY MUFFINS

fun Is there anything better than a freshly baked blueberry muffin? Yes. Two of them!

Makes 12 muffins

1 1/2	cups whole wheat pastry flour
2	teaspoons baking powder
1 1/4	cups coconut sugar
1/4	teaspoon sea salt
1/4	teaspoon allspice
3/4	cup cashew milk
1/4	cup grapeseed or safflower oil
1	large egg
1	teaspoon vanilla extract
1	cup frozen wild blueberries

1. Preheat the oven to 375°F. Grease a 12-cup muffin tin or use paper liners; set aside.

2. In a medium bowl, add the flour, baking powder, coconut sugar, salt, and allspice. Whisk until well blended.

3. Add the milk, oil, egg, and vanilla. Stir until mixture is combined and there are no visible signs of flour. Using a rubber spatula, fold in the blueberries.

4. Evenly spoon the batter into the prepared muffin tin. Bake 25 to 27 minutes, until the muffins spring back when lightly tapped or an inserted metal skewer comes out clean. Let cool at least 10 minutes before serving.

Tia Tip: Folding: This is a specific way of mixing, and it keeps more air in the batter, maintaining lightness. Here's how to fold: Using a rubber spatula, insert it into the center of the batter and fold the batter over itself. Repeat this motion while slowly turning the bowl.

BUCKWHEAT WAFFLES

Cree and I love to make these together, especially on the weekends. FYI: These waffles freeze really well for later use. Just let them cool completely and store them in a resealable plastic bag or airtight container in the freezer. When you're ready to use them, you can just pop them in a toaster—no need to thaw!

Makes six 6-inch-round waffles

1	cup buckwheat flour
1 1/2	cups whole wheat pastry flour
4	teaspoons baking powder
1/2	teaspoon sea salt
1 1/2	cups coconut milk
1	large egg
1/4	cup maple syrup (plus more to serve)
1	teaspoon vanilla extract
1/4	cup coconut oil, melted

1. Preheat your waffle maker.

2. In a medium bowl, combine the flours, baking powder, and salt. Whisk until well mixed. Add the milk, egg, syrup, vanilla, and oil. Whisk until mixture is just combined and there are no visible traces of flour.

3. Ladle the batter into the waffle iron (the amount of batter you use depends on the size of your waffle iron). Cook according to the manufacturer's directions. Serve hot, with additional maple syrup, if desired.

TOFU WESTERN BREAKFAST
WRAP

g-f*

veg

clean

Tofu picks up any flavor that you cook it with, so this dish has some nice strong elements to give the tofu some personality. Soybeans are also ridiculously nutritious.

Serves 4

1	tablespoon extra-virgin olive oil
1	small onion, chopped
1/2	red bell pepper, chopped
1/2	green bell pepper, chopped
	Sea salt to taste
12	ounces extra-firm organic tofu, crumbled
1/2	teaspoon turmeric
	Fresh chopped cilantro to taste (optional)
4	whole wheat or corn tortillas, warmed
	Hot sauce to taste (optional)

I.   In a 10-inch skillet, heat the oil over medium-high heat until shimmering. Add the onion and peppers. Season with salt. Sauté until the vegetables become slightly tender, 2 to 3 minutes. Add the tofu, turmeric, and cilantro to the pan, stirring until well blended.

2.   Spoon an even amount of filling onto the center of each tortilla. Season with some hot sauce, if you're using it. Fold the outer edges of the tortilla over the filling. Cut in half, and serve with additional hot sauce, if desired.

* GLUTEN-FREE IF YOU USE CORN TORTILLAS.

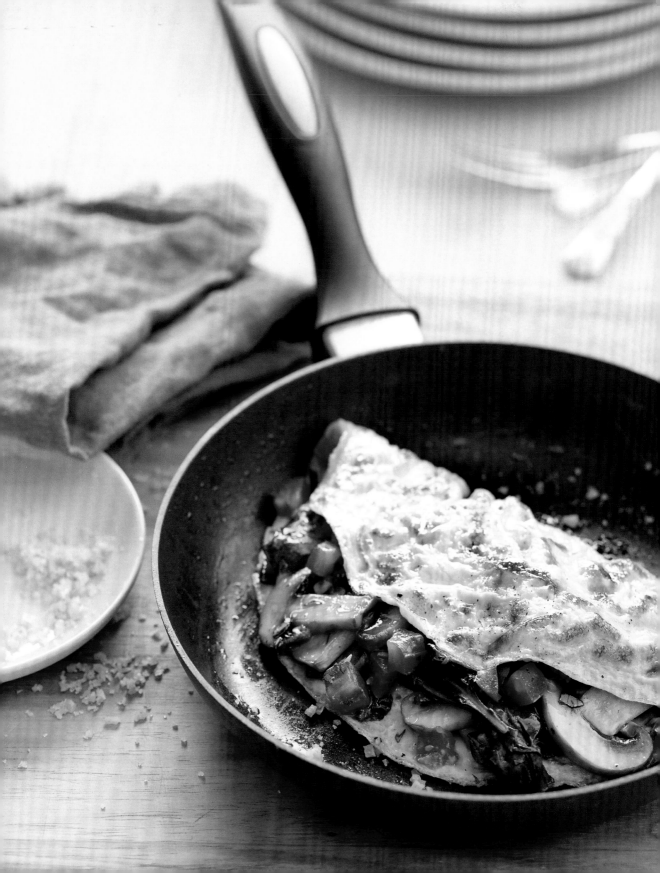

SPINACH, TOMATO, & MUSHROOM OMELET

g-f

clean

Omelets were one of my first dishes as a cook, so I've been practicing for a while now, and these are my best version yet. This is a great breakfast meal, but can be served for dinner, with a big salad. You can also make an egg-white omelet with six egg whites instead of four whole eggs.

Serves 2

- 2 teaspoons extra-virgin olive oil
- 4 ounces white button mushrooms, sliced
- 2 cups packed baby spinach
  Sea salt to taste
- 1 plum tomato, chopped
  Handful of fresh cilantro, chopped
- 4 large eggs, lightly beaten
  Hot sauce, to serve (optional)

1.   In an 8-inch nonstick skillet, heat 1 teaspoon of the oil over medium-high heat until shimmering. Add the mushrooms. Cook, shaking the pan a few times, until the mushrooms are golden, 3 to 4 minutes. Stir in the spinach and season with salt. Cook until just wilted, 1 to 2 minutes. Transfer the vegetables to a bowl. Stir in the tomato and cilantro; set aside.

2.   Heat the remaining teaspoon of oil in the same skillet you used for the vegetables. Season the eggs with salt and pour them into the pan. Cook, without disturbing the eggs, until the edges look set. Use a rubber spatula to lift underneath the edges of the egg, and tilt the pan to let any uncooked egg slide over the edges, to make contact with the skillet and get cooked. Cover one half of the eggs with the vegetable mixture. Fold the plain egg over the half with the vegetables to create a half moon. Cook for 1 minute more. Serve with hot sauce, if desired.

COCONUT, ALMOND, & CRANBERRY GRANOLA

g-f*

veg

Granola is great for breakfast, but it also makes a great snack. Try it on dairy-free yogurt, or just by the handful. *Crunch.*

Makes about 6 cups

4	cups old-fashioned oats (not quick cooking)
1 1/2	cups sliced almonds
1	cup shredded, unsweetened coconut
	Sea salt to taste
1	teaspoon ground cinnamon
1/4	cup extra-virgin olive oil
1/3	cup maple syrup
1	cup fruit-juice-sweetened dried cranberries

1. Preheat the oven to 325°F. Line two 11 x 17-inch rimmed baking sheets with parchment paper.

2. In a deep bowl, combine the oats, almonds, coconut, salt, cinnamon, oil, and syrup. Stir until well mixed. Distribute the mixture between the prepared baking pans.

3. Bake for 30 minutes, stirring halfway through, until the oats and almonds are a deep golden color. Remove the pan from the oven and stir in the dried cranberries. Let the granola cool completely and store it in an airtight container at room temperature for up to 1 week.

* GLUTEN-FREE IF OATS ARE MARKED "GLUTEN-FREE."

SMOOTHIE

g-f

veg

All's fair in love, war, and smoothies. As long as you're combining good-quality ingredients, you really can't go wrong: Add fruit, nut butters, various spices, even vegetables. Go frozen or fresh. Sweet or savory. Explore! I encourage you to experiment and find your favorite combinations. This smoothie is subtle and lovely, with a slightly Indian taste: the perfect springboard for your own creations.

Serves 2

1	cup ripe mango, chopped
1	cup strawberries, topped and halved
1	tablespoon chia seeds
1	teaspoon coconut oil
1	cup unsweetened almond milk
1/2	cup organic apple juice
1/2 to 1	teaspoon ginger juice
1/4	teaspoon cinnamon
1	tablespoon almond butter (optional)

1. Place all ingredients in a blender and blend until smooth. Serve immediately or refrigerate for later.

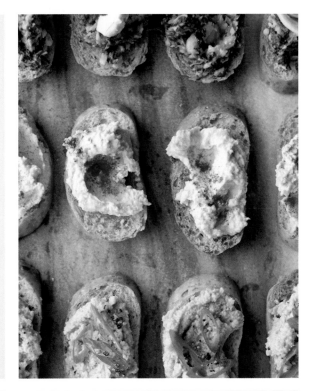

Entertaining

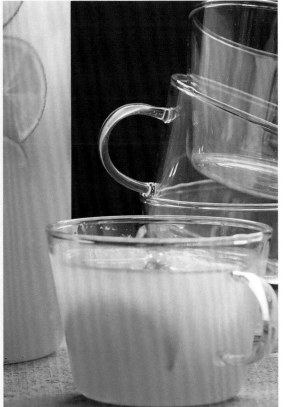

Cory and I like to entertain, and over the years we've come up with some surefire hits to serve to friends and family, no matter their diet. They're delicious and easy and some will get your guests downright tipsy. Have fun!

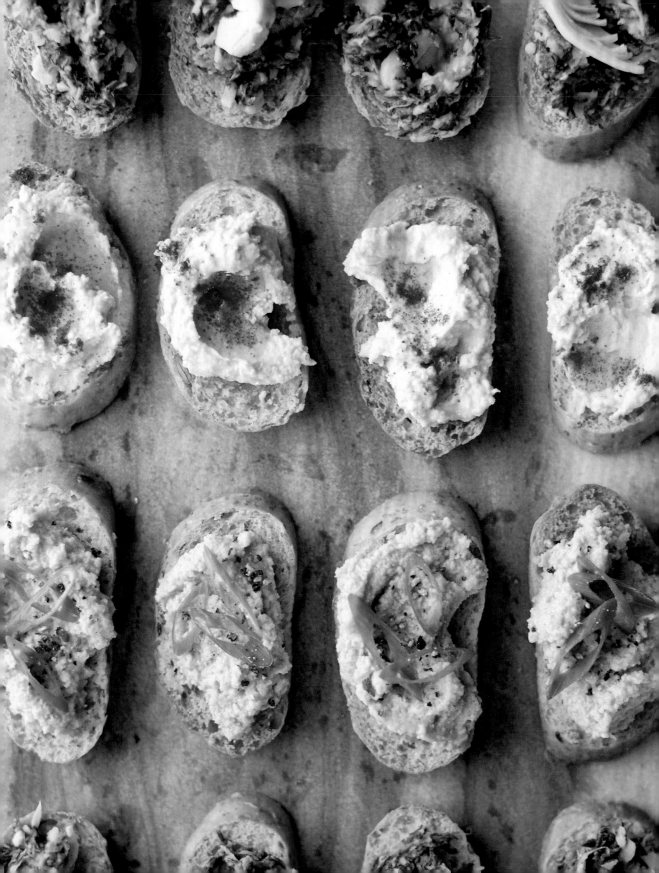

CLASSIC HUMMUS

g-f

veg

clean

Hummus is a great source of protein, complex carbs, and just the right amount of fat. But who cares?!? IT. TASTES. GREAT. I always have hummus on hand because it's the perfect snack for both kids and grown-ups.

Makes about 1 1/2 cups

1	15-ounce can chickpeas, drained and rinsed
3	tablespoons tahini
1	garlic clove
	Freshly squeezed juice of 1 lemon
1/2	teaspoon ground cumin
	Paprika, for garnish
	Extra-virgin olive oil, for garnish

1. In the bowl of a food processor, combine the chickpeas, tahini, garlic, lemon juice, and cumin. Process until it becomes smooth and creamy, drizzling in 2 to 3 teaspoons of water, if needed, to reach the desired consistency. Spread the hummus into a shallow serving dish. Garnish with a few dashes of paprika and a swirl of olive oil before serving. The hummus can be prepared up to 3 days in advance (add the garnish just before serving) and stored in a covered container in the refrigerator.

EDAMAME HUMMUS

Once you've perfected regular hummus, you can explore this different take on it that uses soybeans instead of chickpeas. It's loaded with bold flavors, so the richness of the beans is balanced nicely.

Serves 4

1	10-ounce package frozen organic shelled edamame
1/2	cup water
1	tablespoon soy sauce or tamari
1	tablespoon brown rice vinegar
1	tablespoon toasted sesame oil
1/2	teaspoon minced ginger
1	clove garlic, minced
1/8	teaspoon red chili pepper flakes
1/2	teaspoon sea salt
1	scallion (both green and white parts), thinly sliced

1. Place edamame in a steamer basket in a small pot. Fill pot with water to just under the basket. Sprinkle a pinch of salt over the beans. Cover. Bring to a boil and steam for 20 minutes.

2. Remove from heat and transfer to a dish to cool slightly. Place cooked edamame in a food processor. Add the water, soy sauce (or tamari), vinegar, oil, ginger, garlic, red chili pepper flakes, and salt. Process until smooth. Taste and adjust seasonings, if desired. The scallion can be mixed into the dip or used as a garnish. This is great served with vegetables, on toast, or with rice crackers.

* GLUTEN-FREE IF YOU USE TAMARI.

† [ALTHOUGH RED CHILI PEPPER FLAKES MAY NOT WORK FOR EVERYONE.]

SPINACH & ARTICHOKE DIP

Artichoke dips usually contain some kind of dairy, so I came up with one that's just as tasty but won't leave you feeling like you need to undo the top button of your pants. The cannellini beans give it richness—without the cheese. Serve it on crostini, use it to dip vegetables, or lick it off your fingers!

Makes about 2 1/2 cups

1   cup frozen chopped spinach, thawed
1   14-ounce can artichoke hearts (packed in water)
1   15-ounce can cannellini beans, drained and rinsed
2   garlic cloves
    Freshly grated zest and juice of 1 lemon
1/4 cup extra-virgin olive oil
1/2 teaspoon sea salt, plus more to taste
    Freshly ground black pepper to taste

1.   Place the spinach on a clean kitchen towel. Fold the towel over and squeeze out as much water from the spinach as possible.

2.   In the bowl of a food processor, combine the spinach, artichoke hearts, beans, and garlic. Pulse until it forms a roughly chopped mixture. Add the lemon juice and zest, oil, and salt. Process until smooth and creamy. Season with more salt, if desired, and pepper.

3.   Serve immediately or store in a covered container in the refrigerator for up to 2 days.

CRISPY ROASTED CHICKPEAS

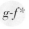

g-f*

veg

clean†

Chickpeas reach a whole new level of flavor when they're roasted. These are great for parties or just for snacking.

Makes about 4 cups

2   15-ounce cans chickpeas, drained and rinsed

3   tablespoons extra-virgin olive oil

1   tablespoon sesame oil

1   tablespoon soy sauce or tamari

1   teaspoon smoked red chili pepper flakes, or more to taste

Flaky sea salt to taste

1. Preheat the oven to 425°F.

2. Remove the skins from the chickpeas and discard. In a deep bowl, combine the chickpeas with the oils and soy sauce (or tamari). Toss until well coated. Spread the chickpeas into a single layer on a 9 x 13-inch rimmed baking sheet.

3. Bake, shaking the pan every 10 to 15 minutes, until the chickpeas are a deep golden brown, 50 to 60 minutes. Immediately transfer the hot chickpeas to a deep bowl. Season with the red chili pepper flakes and salt; toss until well coated. Serve warm, or let cool completely and store in a tightly covered container in a cool dry place for up to 1 week.

Tia Tip: Chickpea Striptease: This recipe works best when the outer skins of the chickpeas have been removed. Here's how: Place the chickpeas on one half of a cloth kitchen towel. Fold the towel over, and roll your hands back and forth over the top of the chickpeas to help loosen their skins. Then take each individual chickpea between your thumb and forefinger and squeeze gently until the chickpea pops out of its skin. Discard the skins. If you don't have time to do this, the recipe will still work, but the result won't be as crispy.

* GLUTEN-FREE IF YOU USE TAMARI.

† [ALTHOUGH RED CHILI PEPPER FLAKES MAY NOT WORK FOR EVERYONE.]

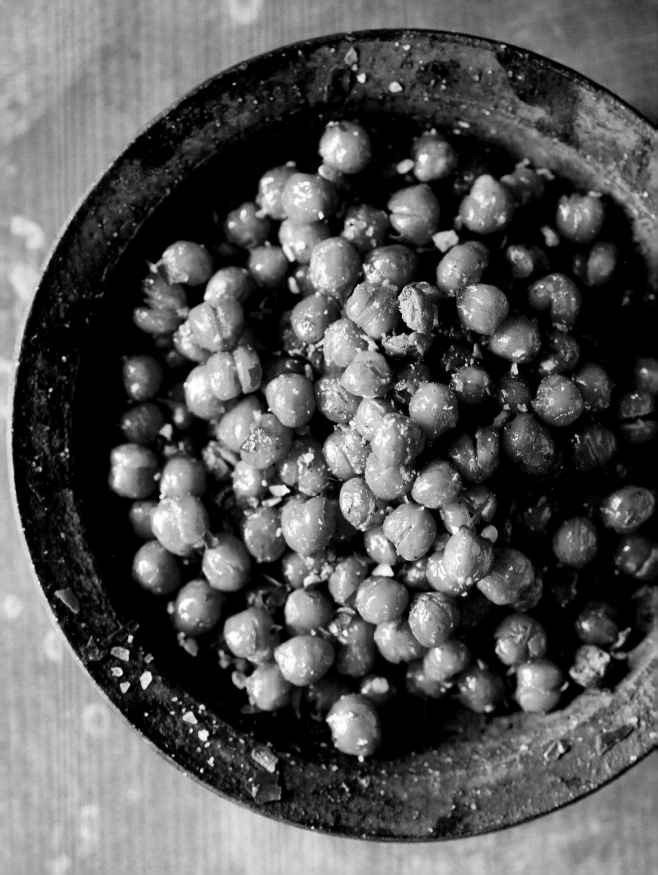

FRIED PICKLES

 fun I was introduced to fried pickles while shooting *The Game* in Atlanta, and they quickly became one of my favorite treats. They taste much naughtier than they are, if you use high-quality ingredients.

Makes 14 pickles

14	1/2-inch-thick round pickle slices
	Safflower oil for frying
1	large egg
1/2	cup coconut milk
3/4	cup whole wheat pastry flour
	Generous pinch of sea salt
1	teaspoon paprika

1. Place the pickle slices in a single layer between two paper towels. Gently pat them dry; set aside.

2. Add 2 inches of oil to a deep pot fitted with a deep-fry thermometer over medium heat. Bring the oil to 375°F.

3. Once the oil reaches 365°F, make the batter. In a deep bowl, combine the egg, milk, flour, salt, and paprika. Whisk until the ingredients are combined and have formed a loose batter.

4. Dip one pickle slice into the batter, shaking off any excess. Carefully drop it into the hot oil. Repeat with a few more pieces (you'll need to do this in batches so as not to crowd the pot, or the pickles will steam and not fry properly). Cook until the pickles are golden underneath, then flip and cook them until they are golden on the other side, about 2 minutes per side.

5. Using a slotted spoon, transfer the pickles to a paper-towel-lined sheet to drain. Serve immediately.

Tia Tip: When it comes to store-bought pickles, it's best to use those that are unpasteurized, organic, and made without sugar. Considering pickles can pack such a healthy punch, why compromise?

PARTY POPCORN

g-f

veg

Impress your guests with this combination of garlic, herbs, and cheesy-tasting nutritional yeast that makes it fun, different, and addictive! This is a riff on a popcorn recipe that's become very popular recently, originally created by Little Lad's, a company based in Maine.

Makes 4 quarts

- 1/2 cup organic popcorn
- 2 tablespoons extra-virgin olive oil
- 1 tablespoon Italian herb mix (usually contains dried versions of basil, marjoram, thyme, sage, oregano, parsley, rosemary—or some combination thereof—and can be purchased pre-mixed)
- 1/4 cup nutritional yeast
- 1/2 teaspoon sea salt
- 1/2 teaspoon garlic powder

1. Pop the popcorn your favorite way and set aside.

2. Heat the olive oil over medium heat until it shimmers. Add the herb mix and remove the pan from the heat. Let the herbs infuse into the oil for 15 minutes. Place the popcorn in a paper bag and drizzle the herbs and oil over it. Close the bag and shake vigorously. Add the nutritional yeast, salt, and garlic powder, and shake some more. Adjust seasonings to taste.

GRILLED "CHEESE" SANDWICH

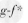

g-f*

veg

fun

Back in the day, dairy-free "cheeses" didn't melt very well. But thanks to the Daiya company, you can now achieve the lovely, stringy melty-ness of real cheese, without dairy or even soy. These sandwiches are great for kids, guests, and hungry husbands.

Makes 4 sandwiches

Extra-virgin olive oil

8   slices whole wheat bread

1   bag Daiya cheddar "cheese" shreds

OPTIONAL EXTRAS:

Pickle slices

Kimchi

Sauerkraut

Grilled Portobello mushroom

Cilantro, chopped

Parsley, chopped

Jalapeño slices

A dollop of pesto

Bacon

Olives

Anything else you can think up!

1.   In a heavy skillet, heat 2 tablespoons of olive oil over medium-low heat. Place 2 slices of bread in the skillet and cover each slice with Daiya cheddar "cheese." Cover the skillet and let the cheese melt. This cheese won't appear (to your eyes) to melt completely, but if you touch it, you'll see that it's soft. When the cheese seems to have melted, remove both slices of bread from the skillet, place them on a plate, and add any optional extras to one slice. Bring the slices together, surrounding the extra ingredients with cheese. Slice and serve.

* GLUTEN-FREE IF YOU USE GLUTEN-FREE BREAD.

BOTTOMS UP!

I'm not a big drinker, but I do like a grown-up beverage every once in a while. People with Candida are supposed to stay away from yeast and sugar so I stick with sake, tequila, and sometimes vodka: They are low in sugar and all the yeasts have been distilled away.

If you really want to discover the power of food (and your body), stay away from all alcohol for a while. If you're in good health, however, an occasional organic beer or glass of wine shouldn't hurt. Although these substances contain simple carbohydrates, they are rich in other nutrients if they're made with good, real ingredients. JUST DON'T DRINK AND DRIVE!!!

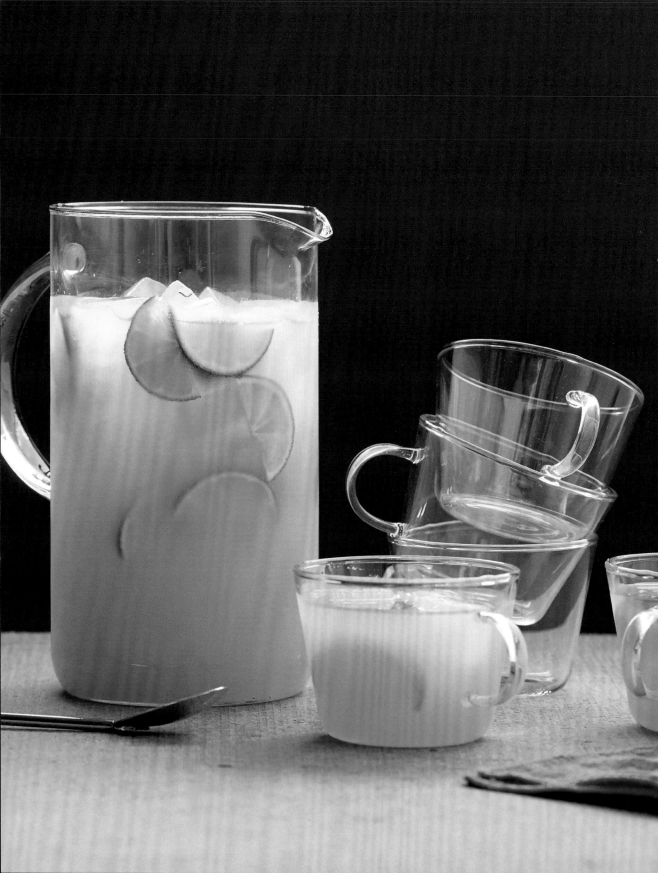

PINEAPPLE GINGER SAKE SANGRIA

g-f

veg

fun

Mix up a batch of this sexy sangria for your next garden party!

Makes 1 quart (serves 8)

2-inch	piece of fresh ginger, peeled and sliced
3	tablespoons agave syrup
2	cups unsweetened pineapple juice
1 1/4	cups sake
1/4	cup freshly squeezed lime juice (from 2 to 3 limes)
	Lime slices, for garnish (optional)

1. In a small pot, mash the ginger to release some of the juices (a bar muddler works great for this, or the back of a wooden spoon). Add the agave syrup. Place the pot on the stove over medium-low heat. Cook until the agave syrup is hot but not boiling. Remove the pot from the heat and let cool completely.

2. Pour the cooled syrup through a fine sieve or strainer; discard the pieces of ginger. Add the agave, pineapple juice, sake, and lime juice to a 1-quart bottle or Mason jar. Seal the bottle closed and shake vigorously to combine ingredients. Chill for at least 4 hours, or overnight.

3. To serve, fill a wine glass to the top with ice and tuck lime slices around the inside of the glass. Pour in sangria, and enjoy!

SAKE MOJITO

g-f

veg

fun

This drink is refreshing and delicious. Perfect for a summer evening. Olé!

Serves 1

2	lime wedges
4	fresh mint leaves
3	drops stevia extract
	Ice cubes
2	ounces sake
	Seltzer

1. Add 1 lime wedge, mint, and stevia to a rocks glass. Use the back of a spoon or a bar muddler to mash the lime wedge and mint leaves. Fill the glass with ice cubes. Pour in the sake. Top off with the seltzer. Stir. Garnish with the remaining lime wedge to serve.

SAKE PIÑA COLADA

g-f

veg

fun

I love coconut milk in drinks. This cocktail will take you on a mini Caribbean holiday!

Serves 4

1	cup unsweetened, crushed pineapple (about half of a 14-ounce can)
1	5.4-ounce can unsweetened coconut cream
3/4	cup sake
12	ice cubes
4	fresh wedges or 4 dried unsweetened slices pineapple, for garnish

1. Add the crushed pineapple, coconut cream, sake, and ice cubes to the bowl of a blender. Pulse until it forms a slushy mixture. Divide among four glasses. Garnish with fresh or dried pineapple, and serve immediately.

Tia Tip: This drink goes *over the top* when the ice cubes in it are made from coconut water! Just freeze the coconut water from the No-Churn Chocolate Espresso Ice Cream recipe (page 267) and use the cubes here or in other drinks.

Make this drink your own by changing up the fruit: Try strawberries, blueberries, raspberries, or a funky combo!

BLACKBERRY MARGARITA

g-f

veg

fun

Serves 1

Ice cubes

1/4   cup frozen blackberries

1¹/₂ ounces tequila

3   ounces sour mix (page 261)

1. Fill a rocks glass halfway with ice. Add the blackberries. Pour in the tequila and sour mix. Stir a few times until well mixed (a chopstick works really well for this!). Serve immediately.

SUGAR-FREE SOUR MIX

Makes 1 1/4 cups

3   limes, juiced

1   lemon, juiced

1   orange, juiced

5   drops stevia extract

I.   Add the juices to a glass Mason jar (you should have about one cup of liquid). Add 1/4 cup of water and the stevia to the jar. Cover tightly with a lid, and shake to combine. Store in the fridge for up to 3 days.

Tia Tip: JUICE THAT LEMON! Before extracting the juice of a lime or lemon, roll the fruit on a counter under the palm of your hand. This ensures that you'll get as much juice as possible.

CRANBERRY DRINK

g-f

veg

fun

When I was on the Body Ecology diet, one of the drinks recommended was cranberry juice, diluted with water (it's strong) and sweetened with stevia. Cranberry juice has a ton of great qualities: It helps treat and prevent urinary tract infections by preventing the growth of bacteria; it contains flavonoids that help lower the risk of heart problems; and its antibacterial properties prevent tooth decay! As if that's not enough, cranberries also help boost immunity and aid digestion. So I drank my cranberry juice.

This next recipe is simple:

1   part cranberry juice
3   parts water
    Stevia to taste

1.   Mix, and serve over ice.

Variation: As my diet opened up, I spiked this drink for parties, adding sake or vodka and lime. Cranberry PARTAY!!!

Desserts

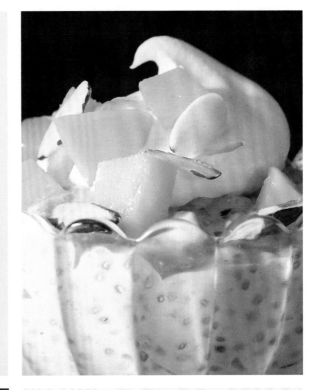

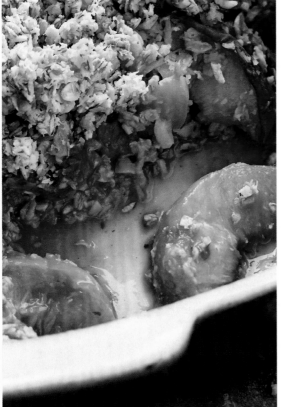

Is it really necessary to introduce a dessert section? If you have the willpower to read this introductory paragraph, your sweet tooth probably isn't as strong as mine. Poor thing.

For the rest of us . . .

Ready . . .

Set . . .

Dessert!

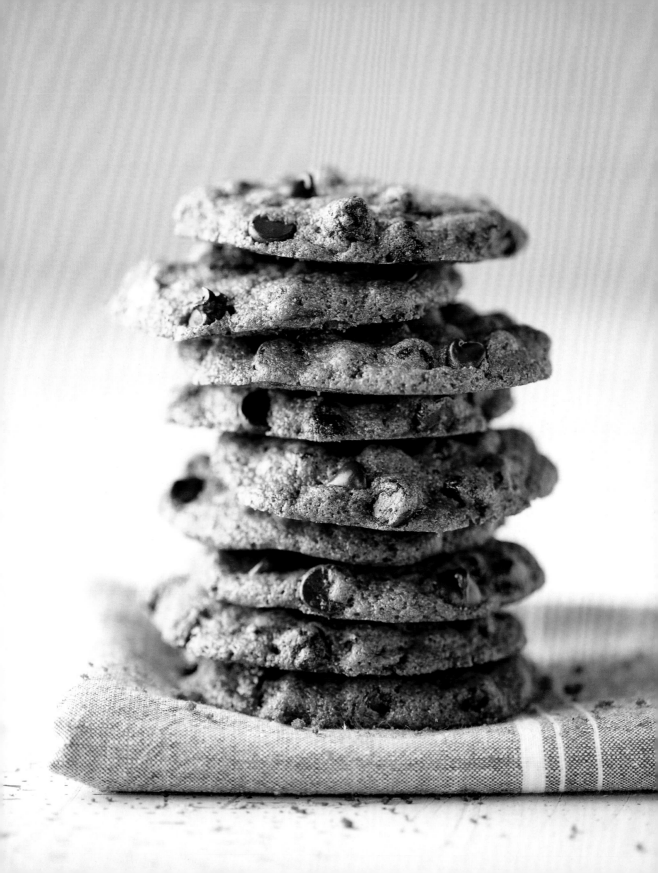

CHEWY CHOCOLATE CHIP COOKIES

 fun These are my favorite. I mean, come on . . . Who doesn't love a chocolate chip cookie?

Makes 45 cookies

1/2	cup safflower oil
1/2	cup coconut sugar
1	large egg (at room temperature)
1	teaspoon pure vanilla extract
1	cup spelt flour or 1 1/4 cups whole wheat pastry flour
1	teaspoon baking soda
1/2	teaspoon sea salt
12	ounces grain-sweetened or stevia-sweetened dairy-free chocolate chips

1. Preheat the oven to 350°F with the rack adjusted to the center position. Line 3 baking sheets with parchment paper (if you have only 2 sheets, just reuse the sheet from the first batch you bake; no need to change the paper).

2. In a deep bowl, combine the oil, sugar, egg, and vanilla. Whisk until smooth and ingredients are incorporated. Add the flour, baking soda, and salt. Stir with a wooden spoon until ingredients are just combined and there are no visible signs of flour. Stir in the chocolate chips.

3. Drop balls of dough (just shy of 1 measured tablespoon each) onto the prepared baking sheets, 2 inches apart (you should be able to fit 15 cookies per sheet). Bake, 1 sheet at a time (it's important for the cookies to bake evenly), until the bottoms and edges are lightly golden and the tops look set, 8 to 9 minutes. Let the cookies cool on the baking sheets for 5 minutes. Use a spatula to transfer them onto a wire rack to cool completely. Store cookies in a covered container for up to 3 days, but they never last that long in my house!

CHEWY FUDGE BROWNIES

fun   These are a household favorite. They disappear in seconds!

Makes 16 1.5-inch-square brownies

6	ounces grain-sweetened or stevia-sweetened dairy-free chocolate chips
2	large eggs
1/4	cup grapeseed or safflower oil
3/4	cup coconut sugar
1	teaspoon vanilla extract
1/4	teaspoon sea salt
1/3	cup whole wheat pastry flour

1.   Preheat the oven to 350°F. Line an 8-inch-square baking pan with a sheet of parchment paper long enough to hang over the sides.

2.   Bring a small pot of water to a boil. Add the chocolate chips to a heatproof bowl that fits snugly over the pot of water. Place the bowl on top of the pot, stirring occasionally, until the chocolate chips are melted; set aside to cool slightly.

3.   Add the eggs, oil, coconut sugar, vanilla, and salt to a deep bowl. Whisk vigorously until well combined. Using a wooden spoon or rubber spatula, stir in the melted chocolate. Add the flour. Stir until ingredients are just combined and there are no visible traces of flour.

4.   Pour the batter into the prepared baking pan. Bake for 18 to 20 minutes, until the tops of the brownies are shiny and they look set in the center. Let cool completely, at least 2 hours, before cutting.

NO-CHURN CHOCOLATE ESPRESSO ICE CREAM

Is there life without ice cream? Of course not. But you don't need the dairy to enjoy it. This recipe is elegant, sexy, and has the built-in pick-me-up of the espresso (use decaf if you plan on eating it right before bedtime!). Chocolate is a natural mood-booster and even an aphrodisiac, so you may have a fun evening ahead!

Makes 1 1/2 pints

2	13.5-ounce cans full-fat coconut milk
12	pitted prunes
1	ounce espresso (single shot)
1	teaspoon vanilla extract
1/4	cup cocoa powder
1	tablespoon maple syrup
	Pinch of sea salt

1. Open the cans of coconut milk and spoon the coconut solids off the top into a deep bowl (save the liquid for another use—see Tia Tip). Using a whisk, beat the coconut solids until they thicken a bit (they won't get super thick like traditional whipped cream, but they'll get a little fluffy); set aside.

2. Add the prunes, espresso, and vanilla extract to the bowl of a food processor. Pulse until it forms a smooth paste.

3. Fold the prune paste, cocoa powder, syrup, and salt into the bowl with the whipped coconut solids.

4. Spoon the mixture into a container, and cover tightly. Freeze for 4 hours, or overnight before serving.

Tia Tip: Got extra coconut milk on hand? After you take the coconut solids off a can of the milk, try freezing the rest of the liquid in an ice cube tray. You can throw the cubes into tropical-tasting drinks, like the one on page 259.

CHOCOLATE-GLAZED VANILLA DOUGHNUTS

 fun Yes, treat yourself to a doughnut! These are delicious, good-looking, and fun to make. The kids will love them, if Mommy doesn't eat them all first.

Makes 6

FOR THE DOUGHNUTS:

3/4	cup whole wheat pastry flour
2	tablespoons coconut sugar
1	teaspoon baking powder
1/4	teaspoon sea salt
6	tablespoons canned coconut cream
1	tablespoon coconut oil, melted
1	large egg
1/2	teaspoon vanilla extract

FOR THE GLAZE:

3	tablespoons coconut cream
2	tablespoons coconut sugar
1/3	cup grain-sweetened or stevia-sweetened dairy-free chocolate chips
1	teaspoon vanilla extract
1	tablespoon brown rice syrup

1. Preheat the oven to 425°F. Coat a 6-slot doughnut pan with cooking spray; set aside.

2. To make the doughnuts: In a medium bowl, combine the flour, coconut sugar, baking powder, and salt. Whisk to blend. Add the coconut cream, coconut oil, egg, and vanilla. Stir with a fork until ingredients are just combined and there are no visible traces of flour.

3. Evenly spoon the batter into the prepared doughnut pan. Bake for 8 to 9 minutes, until the donuts are lightly golden and spring back when touched. Transfer the pan to a wire rack, and let the doughnuts cool completely.

4. Once the doughnuts are cooled, prepare the glaze. Add the coconut cream and sugar to a small pot. Cook over medium-low heat just until the sugar has dissolved (make sure the cream does not come to a boil).

5. Add the chocolate chips to a small, heatproof bowl. Pour the hot cream mixture on top. Add the vanilla. Let sit for 1 to 2 minutes until the chips begin to melt. Stir with a spoon until smooth. Stir in the brown rice syrup. You should have a thick, smooth glaze.

6. Dip the doughnuts into the glaze. Place them on a wire rack, and let stand for a few minutes until the glaze sets.

DARK CHOCOLATE BANANA "MILK" SHAKES

You are not going to believe that this "milk" shake is dairy-free. Everyone will love it!

Serves 4

2   tablespoons nut butter (sunflower, almond, peanut, cashew, etc.)

4   bananas, peeled, cut into pieces and frozen overnight

3/4   cup Coconut Bliss dark chocolate ice cream (or any ice cream made without white sugar)

2   cups plain, unsweetened coconut milk

Unsweetened, shredded coconut, to garnish (optional)

Grain-sweetened or stevia-sweetened chocolate chips to garnish (optional)

1.   Add the nut butter, bananas, ice cream, and coconut milk to a blender. Blend until the mixture is smooth and the banana is completely puréed. Divide among four glasses. Top with shredded coconut and chocolate chips, if desired, before serving.

Tia Tip: There are lots of types of dairy-free ice cream on the market these days—which is fantastic—but they are not all created equal. Be sure to check the label to find out how the ice cream is sweetened. The ones I use contain fruit juice, brown rice syrup, or agave syrup. Sometimes I'll eat the brands made with coconut sugar, but I steer clear of those with cane juice or white sugar.

* GLUTEN-FREE IF YOU USE STEVIA CHOCOLATE CHIPS.

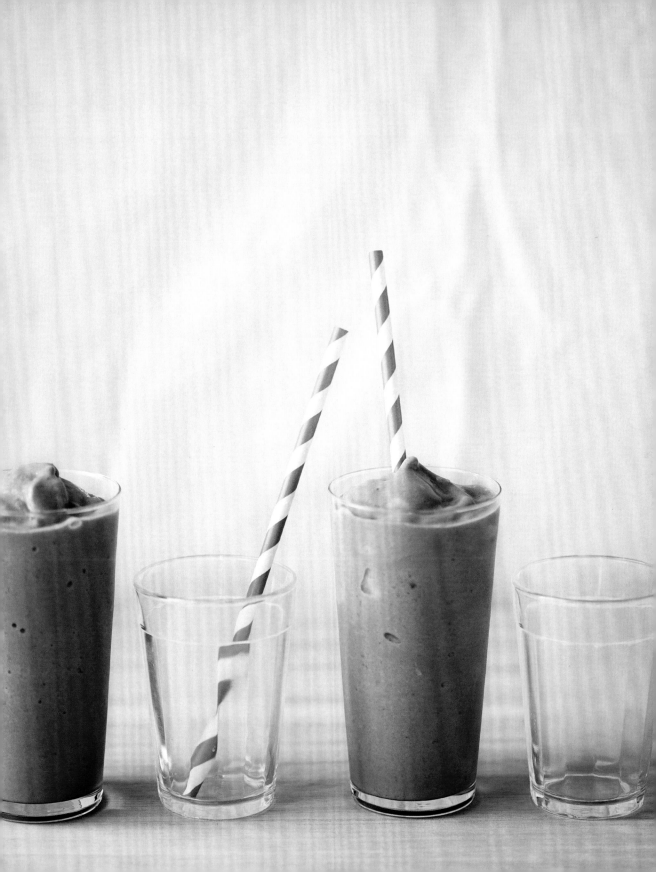

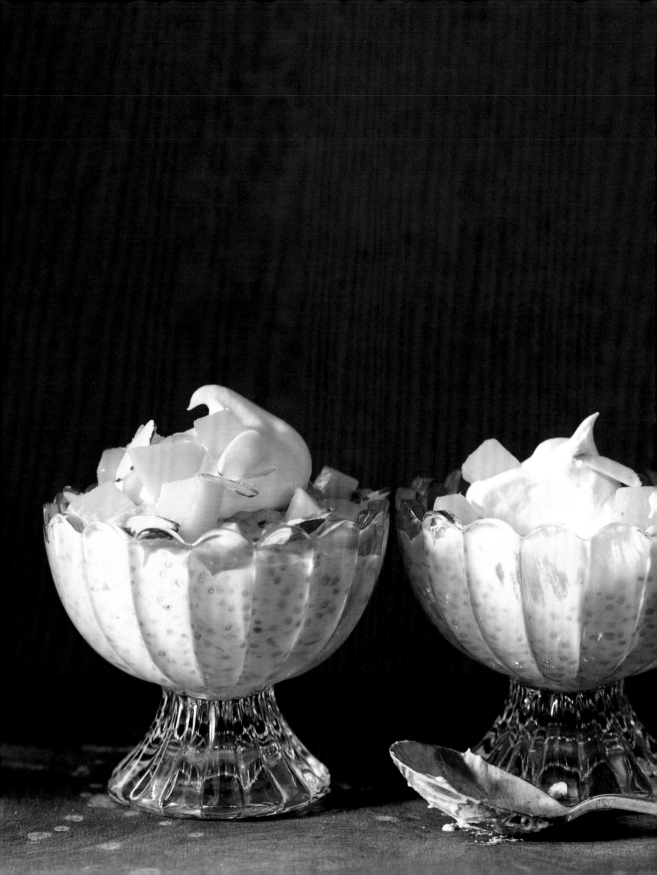

MANGO COCONUT CHIA PUDDING

g-f

veg

Chia seeds are nutritional ninjas. Even though they are tiny and low calorie, they are a great source of omega-3 fatty acids, minerals, fiber, antioxidants, and protein. They also behave in a cool way, becoming sort of gelatinous when they are immersed in fluid. You can find chia seeds at many stores, and they come in either white or black. Although there's no real difference between them nutritionally, you may end up choosing one over the other to achieve a certain look for your recipes.

Serves 4

- 1 cup chopped mango, fresh or frozen (equals 1 fresh mango)
- 1 cup coconut milk
- 1/4 cup agave or maple syrup
- 1/2 teaspoon vanilla extract
- 1/4 cup white chia seeds
- Coconut whipped cream (see Tia Tip)
- 2 tablespoons toasted, sliced almonds, for garnish

1. In a blender bowl, combine the mango and coconut milk. Purée until smooth. Pour into a medium bowl. Add the syrup, vanilla, and chia seeds. Stir until mixed well.

2. Cover the bowl and chill for at least six hours, or overnight. The pudding will keep, covered, for up to 3 days.

3. To serve, spoon into bowls, and top with the coconut whipped cream and almonds.

Tia Tip: Pour just-blended pudding into four Mason jars and refrigerate overnight. Pack (with an ice pack) for a picnic, or in kids' lunches the next morning!

Tia Tip: EASY WHIPPED "CREAM": For quick non-dairy whipped cream, just chill a can of full-fat coconut milk in the fridge overnight. The next morning, open the can and scoop out the solids. With a handheld electric mixer, whip the coconut solids into a lovely whipped cream. You can whip in a few tablespoons of maple or coconut sugar to make it sweeter, if you like.

PEACH RASPBERRY CRISP

g-f*

veg

This is a great summer dessert served with dairy-free ice cream or coconut whipped cream.

Serves 8 to 10

FOR THE TOPPING:

1	cup old-fashioned oats (not quick cooking)
1	cup sliced almonds
1/2	cup shredded, unsweetened coconut
	Pinch of sea salt
3	tablespoons pure maple syrup
1	tablespoon oil (grapeseed or safflower)

FOR THE FRUIT FILLING:

3	ripe peaches, sliced, peeled or unpeeled
1/2	pint fresh raspberries
1/4	cup maple syrup
2	tablespoons fresh-squeezed orange juice (from about 1/2 an orange)

1. Preheat the oven to 375°F.

2. To make the topping: Add the oats, almonds, coconut, and salt to the bowl of a food processor. Pulse until it forms a crumbly mixture. Add the syrup and oil. Pulse 1 to 2 more times until well combined; set aside.

3. Prepare the filling: In a deep bowl, combine the peaches, raspberries, syrup, and orange juice. Stir until well mixed. Spoon the fruit mixture into a 9-inch deep-dish pie plate. Sprinkle the oat mixture over the fruit.

4. Bake 40 to 45 minutes, until the fruit filling begins to bubble and the top is lightly golden. If the topping begins to brown too quickly, cover loosely with a piece of foil. Let the crisp sit on a cooling rack for at least 30 minutes before serving.

* GLUTEN-FREE IF OATS ARE MARKED "GLUTEN-FREE."

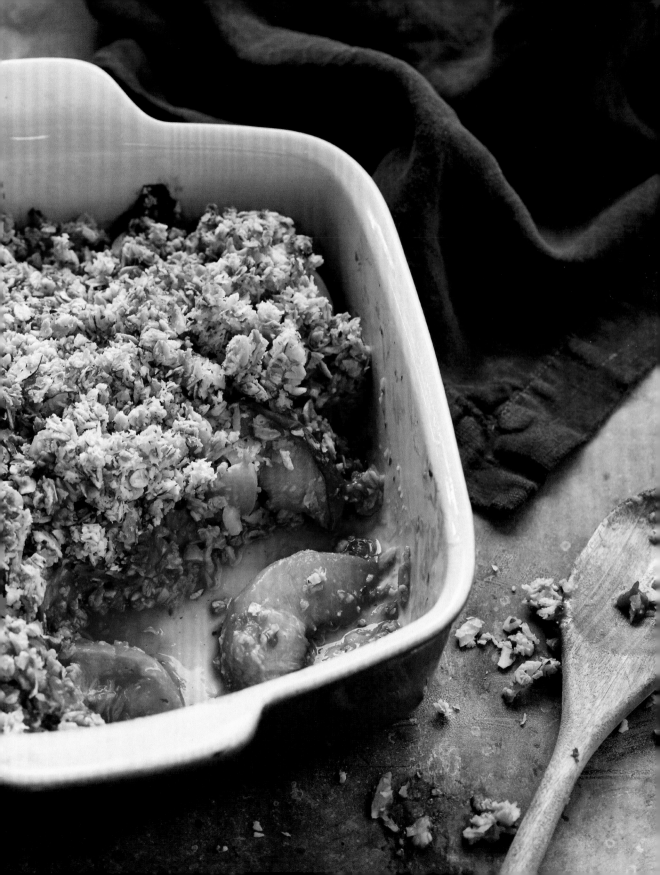

ENERGY BITES

g-f*

veg

clean

These things saved me—and I mean saved me—when I was on a strict detox diet. Mainly, they saved me from looking backward. Whenever I got sugar cravings or felt deprived, I would eat an Energy Bite and all that pain would go away. Plus, they gave me a burst of energy!

Makes 24

1	cup old-fashioned oats (not quick cooking)
1/4	cup shelled hemp seeds
2	tablespoons flaxseed meal
1	tablespoon cocoa powder
1/4	cup shredded coconut, plus more for rolling
	Pinch of sea salt
10	dates, pitted
6	tablespoons almond butter

1. In the bowl of a food processor, pulse the oats until they take on a breadcrumb-like texture. Add the hemp seeds, flaxseed meal, cocoa powder, coconut, and salt. Pulse a few times to combine. Add the dates, and pulse until the whole mixture forms a thick paste. Add the almond butter and pulse a few more times until well combined.

2. Divide the dough into 24 pieces. Roll into balls, and coat with additional shredded coconut, if desired. Store the energy balls in an airtight container in a cool, dry place for up to 1 week.

DESSERTS

* GLUTEN-FREE IF OATS ARE MARKED "GLUTEN-FREE."

CHOCOLATE CAKE *with* CHOCOLATE FROSTING

veg

fun

This. Cake. Rules. No one will guess that it's made without eggs or dairy. It's great for birthday parties, or just because it's Tuesday. YOU'RE WELCOME!

Serves 8

FOR THE FROSTING:

2	cups grain-sweetened chocolate chips (SunSpire is best)
1	cup maple syrup
7	ounces extra firm silken tofu (just over half a box of Mori-Nu brand is good)
	Pinch of sea salt
1	tablespoon vanilla
1	cup soy milk powder

FOR THE CAKE:

1	cup whole wheat pastry flour
1	cup unbleached white flour
2	teaspoons baking powder
2	teaspoons baking soda
1	teaspoon sea salt
1/2	cup plus 2 tablespoons organic cocoa powder
1/2	cup maple sugar
1/2	cup safflower oil
1	cup maple syrup
1	cup unsweetened soy milk
1	cup water
2	teaspoons apple cider vinegar
1	tablespoon vanilla extract

I. Prepare the frosting first. In a double boiler, melt the chocolate chips and maple syrup, stirring occasionally to avoid burning the chocolate. In a food processor, purée the tofu, salt, and

continued on next page

vanilla. Pour the chocolate/maple mixture into the tofu and blend well. Add the soy milk powder, a little bit at a time. Blend well. Let the frosting cool in the fridge while the cake is baking.

2. Preheat oven to 350°F. Prepare two 9-inch cake pans.

3. Sift flour, baking powder, baking soda, salt, 1/2 cup of cocoa powder, and sugar into a large bowl. Stir with a wire whisk to mix.

4. Combine syrup, soy milk, water, vinegar, and vanilla in a second bowl. Mix with a wire whisk until the mixture foams a little. Pour the wet ingredients into the dry and mix until the batter is smooth.

5. Divide the batter into prepared cake pans. Bake on the center rack of the preheated oven for 25 to 30 minutes or until the center of the cake springs back when lightly touched and a toothpick inserted into the center comes out clean. Place the cake pans on wire racks to cool for 10 minutes. Run a knife along the sides of each pan to release the cakes. Turn the cake layers out of the pans directly onto the racks and let cool completely. Frost the top of one layer. Carefully place the second layer on top of the first and frost the top. Using the leftover frosting, cover the sides of the cake.

Tia Tip: Preparing a cake pan: Cake pans are "prepared" so that cakes can slip out of them easily, without getting stuck to the sides of the pan. To prepare a cake pan:

1. Using a pastry brush, lightly paint the pan with a tasteless vegetable oil. I use safflower for this job. You don't need much oil, but make sure the pan gets completely "painted" and that you get into the corners of the pan; that's where cakes get stuck. If you've used too much oil, pour off the excess. The pan should be slippery, but not dripping with oil.

2. Sprinkle a small handful of flour into the pan, and move it around, tapping the sides of the pan lightly so that the flour sticks to the oil all over the pan. Cover it completely, even up the sides of the pan, by turning it on its side and continuing to tap and rotate the pan. Tap out any extra flour that doesn't stick.

3. Voila! You can now pour your cake mix into the prepared pans.

FYI: If you're cooking a chocolate cake and you won't be frosting it (who does that?), substitute cocoa powder for the flour so the finished cake doesn't have a white or beige flour residue.

BERRY "JELL-O" *with* TOPPING

g-f

veg

clean

This recipe uses a type of seaweed called agar agar that creates a very similar consistency to gelatin, but it's much better for you. It's easy and makes a gorgeous dessert. You can find it at any Whole Foods Market or better health-food stores.

Serves 6

FOR THE "JELL-O":

4	cups organic apple juice (set aside 1/2 cup to dilute arrowroot)
1/4	cup rice syrup
	Pinch of sea salt
1/4	cup agar agar flakes
1/4	cup arrowroot starch
1	cup fresh or frozen organic raspberries, halved or roughly chopped

FOR THE CREAMY TOFU TOPPING:

1	pound firm tofu
1	cup rice syrup or 2/3 cup maple syrup
	Pinch of sea salt
1/2	teaspoon vanilla

FOR THE GARNISH:

1/2	cup slivered almonds

1. Bring 31/2 cups of apple juice, rice syrup, salt, and agar agar to a boil. Reduce heat to low and simmer 10 minutes, stirring occasionally until all the agar flakes are dissolved.

2. Dilute the arrowroot in the remaining 1/2 cup of apple juice (this juice must be room temperature or cold in order to dilute the arrowroot properly). Add the arrowroot to the pot, stirring constantly to avoid lumping. As you stir, bring the mixture back to a simmer for about 1 minute. It should thicken slightly and become a little glossy, like a gravy. Add the raspberries and simmer 2 more minutes. Remove from heat and pour into serving cups. Let the pudding set for about 1 hour (refrigeration optional).

3.   Meanwhile, bring a pot of water to a boil. Drop the tofu in and let it cook for 2 minutes. Remove from water. Put the tofu, syrup, salt, and vanilla in a blender or food processor. Whiz ingredients until smooth. Taste and adjust sweeteners to your liking. Chill until cool and slightly thick. When the pudding has set, garnish each serving with a dollop of creamy tofu topping and top with a sprinkle of roasted almonds.

CRISPY RICE TREATS

*g-f**

reg

clean

Rice Krispies treats are a classic dessert, and now you can enjoy a healthier version! This treat will leave you feeling clearheaded, satisfied, and happy. I've never met a person who doesn't like them.

Serves 6 to 8

1	cup brown rice syrup
1/2 to 2/3	cup of your favorite nut butter (I like peanut or almond)
	Pinch of sea salt
	Healthy dash of vanilla
4	cups crispy brown rice cereal

OPTIONAL EXTRAS:

Cinnamon

Nutmeg

Raisins

SunSpire grain sweetened dark chocolate chips, or Lily's stevia-sweetened chocolate chips

Roasted nuts

1. Over a medium flame, heat brown rice syrup, nut butter, salt, and vanilla (and optional cinnamon or nutmeg, if using), stirring constantly until the mixture is smooth, thinned out, and bubbling a little. Reduce heat and let simmer for 3 minutes, stirring constantly.

2. Pour the cereal into a mixing bowl. Add the rice syrup mixture to it and blend well with a wooden spoon. Add optional raisins or nuts, if using. If adding chocolate chips, wait until mixture has cooled a little, so they don't melt completely. Pour into an oiled square pan and flatten with a wet spatula. Let cool. Slice and serve.

* GLUTEN-FREE IF YOU USE LILY'S CHOCOLATE CHIPS.

CITRUS "CHEESECAKE" *with* CHOCOLATE DRIZZLE

g-f*

veg

This is an adaptation of a recipe I found for a dairy-free cheesecake. I've added a chocolate drizzle (have I mentioned I love chocolate?). If you don't like the combination of chocolate and citrus, try the variation.

Serves 8

FOR THE FILLING:

3/4	cup millet, soaked overnight in 2^1/2 cups water
	Pinch of sea salt
3/4	cup cashews, soaked in water to cover overnight and drained in the morning
1/2	cup fresh lime juice (this requires 4 or 5 limes)
1	teaspoon vanilla extract
1/2	cup maple syrup (or ^{1}/4 cup maple syrup and ^{1}/4 cup brown rice syrup, for a slightly less sweet taste)

FOR THE CRUST:

2	cups toasted nuts (almonds, walnuts, or any combination) or 1 cup toasted nuts and 1 cup gluten-free oatmeal
	Pinch of sea salt
4	teaspoons cocoa powder
3/4 to 1	cup pitted dates (soak for 30 minutes if dry, and keep a few extra on hand in case the crust is not moist enough)

FOR THE DRIZZLE:

1	tablespoon cornstarch
3	tablespoons plus ^{1}/8 cup water
1/4	cup fresh lime juice (from 2 to 3 limes)
1/4	cup maple syrup
1	tablespoon unsweetened cocoa powder

continued on next page

* GLUTEN-FREE IF YOU DON'T USE OATS, OR IF OATS ARE MARKED "GLUTEN-FREE."

1.   To prepare the filling: In the morning, cook the millet in the soaking water with a pinch of salt for 45 minutes.

2.   While the millet is cooking, drain the cashews and place them in a blender with lime juice, vanilla, and syrup. Process until very creamy. Set aside and move on to the crust.

3.   To prepare the crust: Grind nuts (or nuts and oatmeal), sea salt, and cocoa powder into a coarse meal in a food processor. Do not overprocess. Add the pitted dates to the nut meal in the food processor while it is running, one date at a time, until the mixture holds together. Press the mixture into the bottom of a 9-inch springform pan.

4.   Return to the filling: When the millet is done, cool it only slightly and add it to the ingredients in the blender (if it cools completely it won't blend well). Process until very, very smooth. Check sweetness and adjust if necessary. Pour the filling into the crust in the pan and let sit for at least 4 hours, unrefrigerated. If you are concerned about dust, or bugs, cover lightly with a breathable cotton tea towel. The "cheesecake" can be refrigerated after it's cool.

5.   Before serving, make the drizzle: Dilute the cornstarch in the 3 tablespoons of water. In a small saucepan, whisk together the rest of the water, lime juice, maple syrup, and cocoa powder. Bring to a boil. Slowly whisk in the cornstarch dilution and stir until it thickens. Drizzle over the whole pie, or individual slices, making fancy designs.

Variation: Skip the cocoa in the crust and use lemon juice instead of lime juice in the filling. Instead of making the drizzle, top the cake with unsweetened, all-fruit jam.

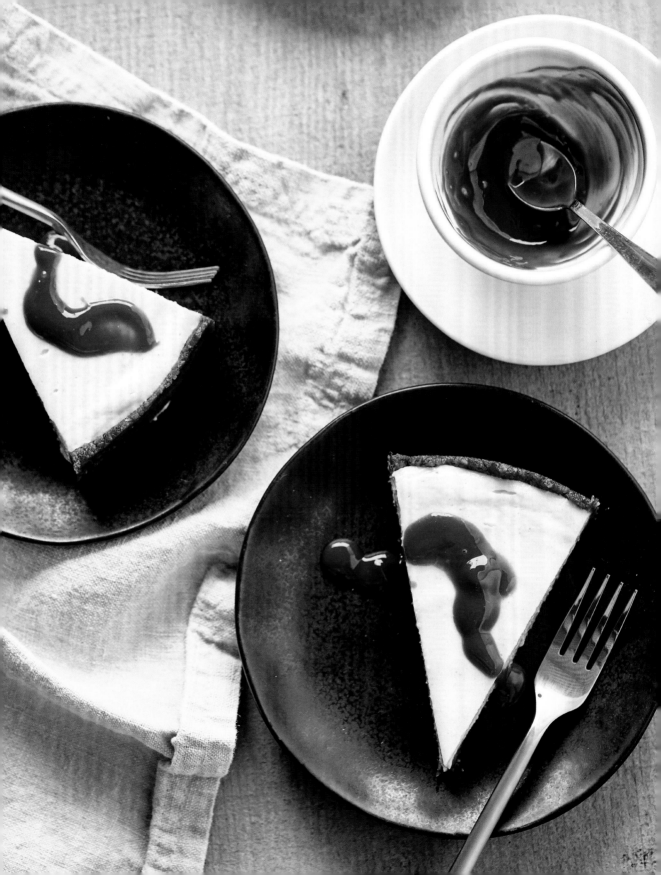

SUMMER SORBET

g-f

veg

clean

The secret is out: It is INCREDIBLY easy to make a good sorbet. Perfect for summer, this dessert satisfies year round.

Serves 4

16   ounces frozen organic raspberries, strawberries, blackberries, or a combination

     Pinch of sea salt

1   teaspoon lemon juice

1/4 cup maple syrup

1.   To make sorbet: Leave the frozen berries out at room temperature for 20 minutes. Then purée them in a food processor until smooth. Add the sea salt, lemon juice, and maple syrup. Process for a few more seconds. Transfer to a freezer container and freeze (up to 2 weeks).

YOUR NEW PANTRY

WHEN I MADE THIS CHANGE TO MY DIET, it was so important for me to remember that I had choices. I wouldn't have been able to let go of white sugar, dairy, and processed foods without knowing that I could eat something equally delicious. Knowing your alternatives is key. This is not a death sentence!

So, instead of buying that cookie from the bakery, I make my own. Instead of a salty Cheeto, I eat savory collard chips. When I am jonesing for dairy, I whip up a nice and gooey grilled non-dairy "cheese" sandwich. You already know some of these ingredients, but I wanted you to have a concrete list of them: hard, documented proof that you will have lovely things to eat. Integrate as many as you can into your cooking, and you are sure to discover a whole new you.

FOOD	WHERE YOU CAN FIND IT/BRANDS
Organic whole grains	Bulk section of Whole Foods Market Bulk section of health-food stores Packaged (especially brown rice) in grocery stores
Organic dried beans	Bulk section of Whole Foods Market Bulk section of health-food stores
Organic canned beans	Many brands, available in most grocery stores and health-food stores
Non-dairy "milks" (almond, oat, rice, soy, hemp, coconut, etc.)	Most grocery stores and health-food stores
Non-dairy sour cream	Recipe on page 163 or Tofutti brand
Non-dairy cream cheese	Tofutti brand
Non-dairy butter	Earth Balance, Smart Balance, and other brands
Non-dairy whipped cream	Recipe on page 273
Non-dairy ice cream	Rice Dream, Almond Dream, Coconut Bliss, So Delicious, Purely Decadent, and other brands
Non-dairy yogurt	So Delicious, Almond Dream, Nancy's, Whole Soy & Co., and other brands
Non-dairy cheese	Daiya, Follow Your Heart, Go Veggie, Rice Vegan, Soy Kaas, Chao, Parmela, Miyoko's Creamery, and other brands
Organic, grass-fed meats	These companies tend to be more local. Look for grass-fed, organic, hormone-free, and antibiotic-free labels. Available at better health-foods stores and Whole Foods Market

FOOD	WHERE YOU CAN FIND IT / BRANDS
Fish	Purchase wild whenever possible
Eggs	Purchase organic. Many brands available
Brown rice syrup	Lundberg, Suzanne's Specialties
Barley malt	Eden Foods
Maple syrup	Many brands available. Grade A is simply lighter than Grade B, not higher in quality
Stevia	Stevia in the Raw, Sweet Leaf, Truvia, and other brands
Coconut sugar	Sweet Tree, Madhava, Now Foods, and other brands
Date sugar	Bob's Red Mill, Chatfields, Now Foods, and other brands
Agave syrup	Madhava, Wholesome Sweeteners, and other brands
Noodles (with gluten)	Look for organic whole wheat, spelt, udon, and/or soba. Many brands available
Noodles (without gluten)	Look for organic rice, quinoa, or corn noodles. Many brands available
Sea vegetables	Available at Whole Foods Market and better health-food stores. Maine Coast Sea Vegetables, Eden Foods, Emerald Cove, Mendocino Sea Vegetable Co.

ACKNOWLEDGMENTS

WRITING A BOOK IS A TEAM EFFORT. I WANT TO THANK, FIRST AND FOREMOST: Cory, Cree, and my whole family. I can do very little without your love and support. You are such great blessings to me.

This book wouldn't exist if Donna Gates hadn't written *The Body Ecology Diet;* it turned my life around in multiple and miraculous ways, for which I will be forever thankful.

I am also grateful to Jessica Porter, who could see my vision from the start and helped me to get it all down on paper. Jennifer Perillo helped to develop and test many of the recipes, which are utterly fantastic, and Jennifer Davick took the gorgeous photos of them. Elizabeth Messina took the lovely family photos of me, Cory, and Cree. I am extremely thankful to you all for your fine talent and hard work.

Thanks to Katherine Latshaw, my wonderful literary agent at Folio, and the kick-ass ladies at Ballantine Books, Nina Shield and Sara Weiss. Thank you all for choosing to bring this project to life. And finally, I am grateful to Ryan Bundra and Adam Griffin for always bringing my visions to fruition.

NOTES

1. Monte Morin, "Organic Foods Are More Nutritious, According to Review of 343 Studies," *Los Angeles Times*, July 14, 2014, http://www.latimes.com/science/la-sci-organic-foods-20140715-story.html.

2. https://www.hsph.harvard.edu/news/press-releases/whole-grains-lower-mortality-rates/.

3. Bahar Gholipour, "Diet High in Meat Proteins Raises Cancer Risk for Middle-Aged People," *Scientific American,* March 4, 2014, http://www.scientificamerican.com/article/diet-high-in-meat-proteins-raises-cancer-risk-for-middle-aged-people/. "Meat Consumption and Cancer Risk," Physicians Committee for Responsible Medicine, http://www.pcrm.org/health/cancer-resources/diet-cancer/facts/meat-consumption-and-cancer-risk.

4. Eliza Barclay, "Eating to Break 100: Longevity Diet Tips from the Blue Zones," *The Salt,* http://www.npr.org/sections/thesalt/2015/04/11/398325030/eating-to-break-100-longevity-diet-tips-from-the-blue-zones.

5. Christelle Devillé, Myriam Gharbi, Guy Dandrifosse, and Olivier Peulen, "Study on the Effects of Laminarin, a Polysaccharide from Seaweed, on Gut Characteristics," *Journal of the Science of Food and Agriculture* 87: 9, 1717–25, July 2007.

6. Hiromitsu Watanabe, "Beneficial Biological Effects of Miso with Reference to Radiation Injury, Cancer and Hypertension," *Journal of Toxicologic Pathology* 26: 2, 91–103, June 2013, http://www.ncbi.nlm.nih.gov/pmc/articles/PMC3695331/.

7. I. Deniņa, P. Semjonovs, A. Fomina, R. Treimane, and R. Linde, "The Influence of Stevia Glycosides on the Growth of Lactobacillus Reuteri Strains," *Letters in Applied Microbiology* 58: 3, 278–84, March 2014, http://www.ncbi.nlm.nih.gov/pubmed/24251876.

8. Hilary Parker, "A Sweet Problem: Princeton Researchers Find that High-Fructose Corn Syrup Prompts Considerably More Weight Gain," March 22, 2010, http://www.princeton.edu/main/news/archive/S26/91/22K07/.

9. Kimber L. Stanhope et al., "Consumption of Fructose and High Fructose Corn Syrup Increase Postprandial Triglycerides, LDL-Cholesterol, and Apolipoprotein-B in Young Men and Women," *Journal of Clinical Endocrinology and Metabolism* 96: 10, E1596–E1605, October 2011, http://www.ncbi.nlm.nih.gov/pmc/articles/PMC3200248/.

10. Kathleen A. Page et al., "Effects of Fructose vs Glucose on Regional Cerebral Blood Flow in Brain Regions Involved With Appetite and Reward Pathways," *Journal of the American Medical Association* 309: 1, 63–70, January 2013, http://jama.jamanetwork.com/article .aspx?articleid=1555133.

11. Richard J. Johnson et al., "Potential Role of Sugar (Fructose) in the Epidemic of Hypertension, Obesity and the Metabolic Syndrome, Diabetes, Kidney Disease, and Cardiovascular Disease," *American Journal of Clinical Nutrition* 86: 4, 899–906, October 2007, http://ajcn .nutrition.org/content/86/4/899.full#sec-10.

12. Roberto A. Ferdman, "Where People Around the World Eat the Most Sugar and Fat," *Washington Post*, February 5, 2015, http://www.washingtonpost.com/news/wonkblog/wp/2015/ 02/05/where-people-around-the-world-eat-the-most-sugar-and-fat/.

13. Nolan Feeney, "Illegal Antibiotics Could Be in Your Milk, FDA Finds," *Time*, March 9, 2015, http://time.com/3738069/fda-dairy-farmers-antibiotics-milk/.

14. 15 http://www.ncbi.nlm.nih.gov/books/NBK44624/#ch3.s1.

15. 16 https://ghr.nlm.nih.gov/condition/lactose-intolerance#inheritance.

16. David M. Hegsted, "Calcium and Osteoporosis?," *Advances in Nutritional Research* 9, 119–28, 1994.

17. http://researchsubmission.nationaldairycouncil.org/HowItWorks/Pages/FundingOppurtu-nities.aspx#GeneralSolicitation. Italics added.

18. http://researchsubmission.nationaldairycouncil.org/HowItWorks/Pages/FundingOppurtu-nities.aspx#GeneralSolicitation. Italics added.

19. http://jn.nutrition.org/content/128/6/1051.full.

20. Kazumi Maruyama, Tomoe Oshima, and Kenji Ohyama, "Exposure to Exogenous Estrogen through Intake of Commercial Milk Produced from Pregnant Cows," *Pediatrics International* 52: 1, 33–8, February 2010.

21. William J. Cromie, "Growth Factor Raises Cancer Risk," *Harvard University Gazette*, April 22, 1999, http://news.harvard.edu/gazette/1999/04.22/igf1.story.html.

22. Antonis Zampelas, Demosthenes B. Panagiotakos, Christos Pitsavos, Christina Chryso-hoou, and Christodoulos Stefanadis, "Associations between Coffee Consumption and In-flammatory Markers in Healthy Persons: The ATTICA Study," *American Journal of Clinical Nutrition* 80: 4, 862–7, October 2004, http://ajcn.nutrition.org/content/80/4/862.full.

23. "Consumer Trends: 83 Percent of Americans Drink Coffee," Food Manufacturing, April 8, 2013, http://www.foodmanufacturing.com/news/2013/04/consumer-trends-83-percent-americans-drink-coffee.

24. Daniel Costa-Roberts, "Fast Food Kills Gut Bacteria that Can Keep You Slim, Book Claims," PBS NewsHour, May 10, 2015, http://www.pbs.org/newshour/rundown/junk-food-kills-helpful-gut-bacteria-study-finds/.

25. http://www.businessinsider.com/americans-are-drinking-less-soda-2016-3.

26. Michael Moss, "The Extraordinary Science of Addictive Junk Food," *New York Times*, February 20, 2013, http://www.nytimes.com/2013/02/24/magazine/the-extraordinary-science-of-junk-food.html?_r=0.

27. "Food Industry Pursues the Strategy of Big Tobacco" (interview with Kelly Brownell), *Yale Environment 360*, April 8, 2009, http://e360.yale.edu/feature/food_industry_pursues_the_strategy_of_big_tobacco/2136/.

28. http://www.ucsusa.org/sites/default/files/legacy/assets/documents/food_and_agriculture/cafos-uncovered.pdf.

29. Christopher D. Heaney, Kevin Myers, Steve Wing, Devon Hall, Dothula Baron, and Jill R. Stewart, "Source Tracking Swine Fecal Waste in Surface Water Proximal to Swine Concentrated Animal Feeding Operations," *Science of the Total Environment* 511, April 1, 2015, 676–83, http://www.ncbi.nlm.nih.gov/pubmed/25600418.

30. http://www.sierraclub.org/michigan/cafo-facts#health-effects.

31. http://www.nmfs.noaa.gov/aquaculture/faqs/faq_feeds.html#1.

32. 32 http://naturalsociety.com/cows-eat-6-surprising-things-fed-us-cows/.

33. ttp://www.npr.org/sections/thesalt/2012/09/06/160684126/why-we-rarely-feed-animals-food-scraps-even-in-a-drought.

34. Aaron Smith, "Cash-Strapped Farmers Feed Candy to Cows," CNNMoney, October 10, 2012, http://money.cnn.com/2012/10/10/news/economy/farmers-cows-candy-feed/.

35. Jorge Fernandez-Cornejo, Seth Wechsler, Mike Livingston, and Lorraine Mitchell, "Genetically Engineered Crops in the United States," Economic Research Report No. 162, Economic Research Service, U.S. Department of Agriculture, February 2014, http://www.ers.usda.gov/media/1282246/err162.pdf.

36. Beth Hoffman, "GMO Crops mean More Herbicide, Not Less," *Forbes*, July 2, 2013, http://www.forbes.com/sites/bethhoffman/2013/07/02/gmo-crops-mean-more-herbicide-not-less/.

37. https://www.usda.gov/oig/webdocs/24601-08-KC.pdf.

38. T. Colin Campbell and Thomas Campbell, *The China Study*, Dallas, TX: BenBella Books, 2004, p. 165.

39. http://www.fda.gov/downloads/ForIndustry/UserFees/AnimalDrugUserFeeActADUFA/UCM440584.pdf.

40. http://www.fda.gov/downloads/drugs/drugsafety/informationbydrugclass/ucm319435.pdf.

41. http://www.sciencedirect.com/science/article/pii/S1687428513001167.

42. Monica Eng, "Another Concern: Drug Residues in Meat," *Chicago Tribune*, May 26, 2013, http://articles.chicagotribune.com/2013-05-26/news/ct-met-antibiotics-residue-20130526_1_u-s-meat-the-fda-drug-violations.

43. George Washington University Milken Institute School of Public Health, "Retail Meat Is a

Potential Vehicle for Disease-Causing Klebsiella," ScienceDaily, July 23, 2015, http://www
.sciencedaily.com/releases/2015/07/150723083723.htm.

44. "California Brings in Strict Limits on Use of Antibiotics in Livestock Farming," *The Guardian,*
October 11, 2015, https://www.theguardian.com/us-news/2015/oct/11/california-brings-in-
strict-limits-on-use-of-antibiotics-in-livestock-farming.

45. Stephanie Strom, "Perdue Sharply Cuts Antibiotic Use in Chickens and Jabs at Its Rivals,"
New York Times, July 31, 2015, http://www.nytimes.com/2015/08/01/business/perdue-and-
the-race-to-end-antibiotic-use-in-chickens.html?_r=0.

46. http://www.fda.gov/AnimalVeterinary/SafetyHealth/ProductSafetyInformation/
ucm055436.htm.

47. Marina Hidalgo, Isabel Prieto, Hikmate Abriouel, Antonio Cobo, Nabil Benomar, Antonio
Gálvez, and Magdalena Martínez-Cañamero, "Effect of Virgin and Refined Olive Oil Consumption on Gut Microbiota. Comparison to Butter," *Food Research International* 64, October 2014, 553–9, http://www.sciencedirect.com/science/article/pii/S0963996914005079.

48. Nicola Wilck, Scott Olesen, Mariana Matus, Andras Balogh, Ralf Dechend, Eric Alm, and
Dominik Muller, "Abstract 321: A High-Salt Diet Alters the Composition of Intestinal Microbiota in Mice," American Heart Association, *Hypertension* 64, 2014, A321, http://hyper.aha
journals.org/content/64/Suppl_1/A321.abstract.

INDEX

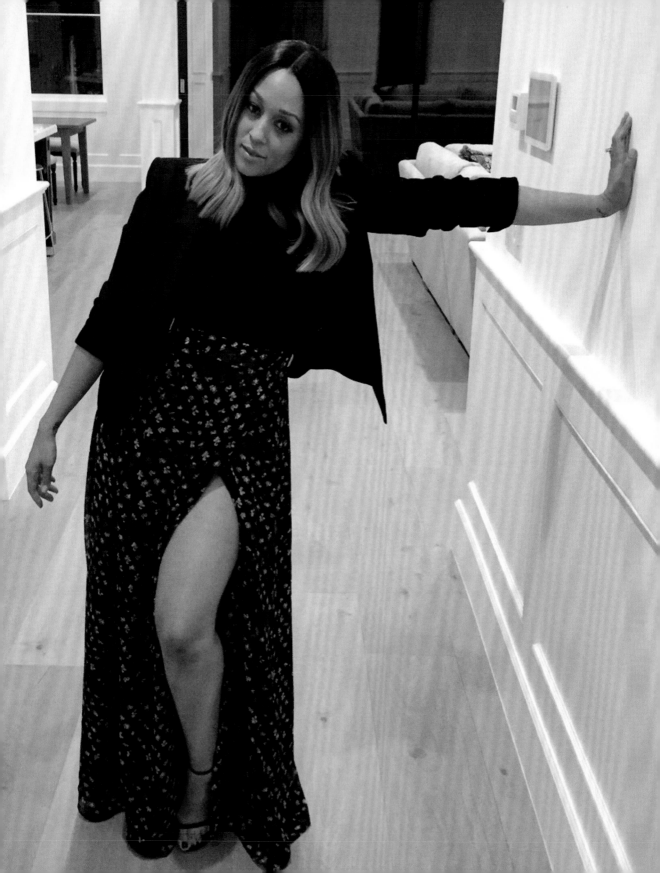

ABOUT THE AUTHORS

TIA MOWRY-HARDRICT has been in the public eye for more than twenty years, gaining initial fame in her teens starring opposite her twin sister in the hit comedy *Sister, Sister.* Her work on the series won her two NAACP Image Awards for Outstanding Actress in a Comedy Series, and three Kids Choice Awards for Favorite Television Actress. After the series wrapped production, Mowry attended Pepperdine University, where she graduated with a bachelor's degree in Psychology. In 2013 Mowry published her debut book, *Oh, Baby!: Pregnancy Tales and Advice from One Hot Mama to Another;* and she is currently rolling out a middle-grade series, *Twintuition,* that she cowrote with her sister. Tia recently wrapped up the second season of her hit show *Tia Mowry at Home* for the Cooking Channel. She is also known for her lead role on The CW/BET's hit show *The Game,* as well as the Nickelodeon series *Instant Mom.* When not acting, she spends time in Los Angeles with her husband, actor Cory Hardrict, and her son, Cree Taylor.

JESSICA PORTER lives and writes in Los Angeles. She is the author of *The Hip Chick's Guide to Macrobiotics* and *The MILF Diet.* When she's not eating, Jessica loves inspiring others to make healthy food choices.